Methylene Blue

A Comprehensive Guide to Breakthrough
Treatments for Modern Times

Braithwaite J. Cooks

Acknowledgement

I want to sincerely thank everyone who has helped me along the way in my career, especially my friends, family, mentors, and coworkers. I have been able to accomplish my goals and make significant contributions to the medical world because of your unfailing support and belief in my talents. Without your love and support, this book would never have happened. I'm grateful.

Furthermore, I want to express my gratitude to all of the researchers, doctors, and patients whose experiences and insights have helped me to better understand methylene blue and its possible therapeutic uses. My goal is that this thorough guide will be an invaluable tool for anybody interested in learning more about this intriguing substance and its potential applications in contemporary medicine, regardless of background knowledge.

About the Author

Braithwaite J Cooks is a renowned scientist and researcher, an expert in molecular biology and neurology. She graduated from Stanford University with a Ph.D. in biochemistry and finished her postdoctoral studies at Harvard Medical School. Several scientific studies written by Braitwhite have been published in esteemed magazines including Cell, Science, and Nature. Her ground-breaking research on Methylene blue as a cutting-edge treatment for a range of diseases has won her praise and recognition on a global scale.

In addition to her career achievements, Braitwhite is an enthusiastic runner and hiker who loves the great outdoors. She also instructs poor children in science as a volunteer at neighborhood community centers. She wants to encourage the next generation of scientists to work in fields devoted to finding creative answers to urgent medical issues through her writing and advocacy work.

Table of Contents

Introduction

For almost 200 years, methylene blue (MB) has been used in several industrial and medicinal settings. Since its first synthesis in 1876, MB has shown itself to be a flexible substance with a range of medicinal applications. Although methemoglobinemia, a disorder marked by abnormally high blood levels of the protein, is the main reason for MB's recognition, it has recently attracted a lot of attention because of its potential uses in treating a variety of diseases.

Because of its distinct combination of qualities, MB is a desirable candidate for therapeutic development. Because it is a tiny molecule, it may easily pass through cell membranes and enter many kinds of cells and tissues. Furthermore, MB can regulate a number of cellular processes, such as inflammation, oxidative stress, and mitochondrial function, which supports its potential use as a treatment in a range of diseases.

With a focus on its potential as a neuroprotective agent in neurological disorders, anxiolytic and antidepressant in depression and anxiety disorders, protective in stroke and traumatic brain injury, antimicrobial, anti-cancer, and other emerging therapeutic potentials, the current article aims to provide an overview of the diverse therapeutic applications of MB. The underlying processes and supporting data for MB's therapeutic potential in each application will be thoroughly discussed in each section.

The Background Of Methylene Blue In History

Synthetic compounds like methylene blue (MB) have a long history that dates back to the middle of the 1800s. German scientist Heinrich Caro, who was employed at the Badische Anilin- und Soda-Fabrik (BASF) firm, created the substance for the first time in 1876. After preliminary testing revealed that MB could be used as a dye for silk and cotton textiles, the textile industry widely adopted it.

When German scientist and physician Paul Ehrlich, who was awarded the Nobel Prize in 1891, realized that MB could stain live cells, he gave it the moniker "selective vital dye." Its usage as a diagnostic tool in medicine, especially in the field of hematology, was prompted by this finding, and it is now a routine test for identifying aberrant hemoglobin variations.

When MB was used to treat a patient with methemoglobinemia, a disorder marked by excessively high amounts of methemoglobin in the blood, the medicinal potential of the substance was first recognized in 1899. Since then, MB has been utilized in medicine to treat a range of conditions, including cyanide poisoning, malaria, and urinary tract infections.

MB was utilized as a local anesthetic, antipyretic, and antimalarial medication in the early 1900s. However, the availability of more modern and potent medications caused its usage to wane in the second half of the 20th century. However, there has been a resurgence of interest in MB's therapeutic potential recently, especially in the domains of cancer and neurosciences, where its neuroprotective and antitumor properties have been shown.

The US Food and Drug Administration (FDA) has authorized MB as a medication for the treatment of methemoglobinemia, and it is currently obtainable as a prescription medication under several brands. Even though MB has been used for a long time, research into its medicinal potential is always continuing, and novel uses are always being investigated. The chemical is a promising candidate for repurposing as a therapeutic agent for a variety of medical problems due to its distinct qualities and adaptable modes of action.

Contemporary Research and Applications

Methylene blue (MB) has garnered renewed attention as a possible therapeutic agent for a number of ailments in recent years. This is partially explained by the discovery of its many, adaptable mechanisms of action, which include, among other things, neuroprotective, anti-inflammatory, and antioxidant properties.

The study of neurology is among the most exciting fields of MB research. It has been demonstrated that MB has neuroprotective benefits in a number of neurological conditions, such as stroke, Parkinson's disease, and Alzheimer's disease. One possible explanation for its neuroprotective properties has been proposed: it can modify mitochondrial activity and minimize oxidative stress.

Moreover, MB has demonstrated potential in the treatment of anxiety and depression. According to a number of studies, MB helps people with major depressive disorder, bipolar disorder, and post-traumatic stress disorder feel less depressed and anxious. Though the precise mode of action is unknown, monoaminergic neurotransmitters like dopamine and serotonin are thought to be modulated.

Other diseases where MB has demonstrated potential as a therapeutic agent include stroke and traumatic brain injury. In animal models of stroke and traumatic brain damage, MB has been demonstrated to lower oxidative stress and inflammation, indicating that it may have neuroprotective benefits in these situations.

MB's antibacterial qualities have also been studied. It is a possible contender for the creation of novel antimicrobial medications because of its demonstrated antiviral, antifungal, and antibacterial properties.

In several cancer cell lines and animal models, MB has demonstrated anti-cancer properties in the field of oncology. Its anti-cancer actions may be attributed to its capacity to alter mitochondrial activity and cause apoptosis in cancer cells.

Additional therapeutic uses for MB include treating skin diseases including eczema and psoriasis, treating alcohol use disorder, and acting as a photosensitizer in photodynamic therapy.

Larger, more carefully planned clinical trials are still required to confirm the safety and effectiveness of MB as a therapeutic agent for a range of medical problems, even in light of the encouraging findings from preclinical research. However, an increasing amount of data points to MB's potential as a useful therapeutic drug with a variety of medicinal uses.

The Goal And Extent Of The Book

This book aims to give a thorough overview of the therapeutic uses of methylene blue (MB), a chemical with a wide range of uses and historical significance that has been employed in both industrial and medicinal settings for more than a century. Researchers, physicians, students, and everyone else with an interest in learning about the most recent advancements in MB research and its possible therapeutic applications should find this book to be a useful resource.

The book covers the chemistry, pharmacology, and mechanisms of action of MB from a historical standpoint. In addition to its usage in neurological diseases, depression and anxiety disorders, stroke and traumatic brain damage, antibacterial characteristics, and anti-cancer activities, the book concentrates on the most promising therapeutic applications of MB. The book also delves into additional recently discovered therapeutic applications of MB, including its use in retinal diseases and wound repair.

Experts in the area have authored each chapter of the book, which offers a thorough overview of the status of the literature, clinical uses, and potential future developments for each medicinal use of MB. Tables, figures, and references are also included throughout the chapters to facilitate comprehension and interpretation.

A review of MB's drawbacks and restrictions as a therapeutic agent, including possible toxicity, medication interactions, and pharmacokinetics, is included in the book's conclusion. The potential for more study and cooperation in the area of MB research and its therapeutic applications is also highlighted in the book.

The overall goal of this book is to offer a thorough and reliable resource on the medicinal uses of methylene blue, highlighting the drug's potential as a useful treatment for a range of diseases.

Sources and Methods

Writing this book required a thorough analysis of the body of research on methylene blue's medicinal uses. Information was gathered from both primary and secondary sources, including books, conference proceedings, research publications, review papers, and patents. Relevant keywords and phrases, such as "methylene blue," "therapeutic applications," "neuroprotection," "antineoplastic," "antibacterial," and "antiviral," among others, were used to search online databases including PubMed, Web of Science, Scopus, and Google Scholar.

English language, publication date within the previous 20 years, and topic relevance were the inclusion criteria used to choose the sources. For the purpose of presenting a fair and impartial assessment of the current status of methylene blue research and therapeutic uses, the chosen sources were carefully examined and combined. Preference was always given to excellent, peer-reviewed publications that were published in respectable journals.

In order to add to the literature study and offer knowledgeable thoughts and insights, the writers also relied on their own experience and competence in the subject. Subject matter experts and experienced editors examined and revised the content to make sure it was accurate, clear, and consistent.

Overall, a thorough and rigorous search of the literature, a critical analysis and synthesis of the available clinical and research data, as well as expert opinion and commentary, comprised the approach used for this work. The intention was to offer a thorough and authoritative resource on methylene blue's therapeutic uses, encompassing both well-established and recently-discovered fields of study.

Fundamentals of
Methylene Blue

Chemistry and Pharmacology

Structural Formula and Properties

Methylene blue is a member of the phenothiazines class of chemical compounds, which are characterized by the bridgehead position of a diphenylamine being replaced with a sulfur atom. A core benzene ring is joined to two five-membered rings in the structural formula of MB; one of these rings is fused to a second benzene ring and has a nitrogen atom in it. One of the five-membered rings has a carbonyl group linked to it, while the center benzene ring has two dimethylamino groups attached to it

MB has a molar mass of 319.85 g/mol and the chemical formula C16H18ClN3S. The crystalline powder known as MB has a little solubility in ethanol and water, but it dissolves more readily in diluted mineral acids. It breaks down at temperatures higher than 350°C and has a melting point of 298°C. Under normal circumstances, MB is stable, although it can react with strong bases and oxidizing agents.

Pharmacological

MB is a weak base that, depending on the pH of its environment, can exist in either its unionized or ionized state. MB is mostly found in its unionized form at physiological pH, which is around 7.4. This form is easily able to pass through biological membranes and enter cells. Because MB may ionize and take up protons inside of cells, it accumulates in acidic areas like mitochondria and lysosomes.

The therapeutic benefits of MB are attributed to many modes of action. Being an electron carrier—accepting electrons from substrates and transmitting them to electron acceptors is one of its main functions. Because of this characteristic, MB can participate in redox processes that are essential to cellular metabolism and energy generation, acting as a redox mediator.

Additionally, several enzymes involved in signal transduction pathways, such as guanylate cyclase and nitric oxide synthase, can be inhibited by MB. MB may modify the activity of several signaling molecules, including as cAMP, cGMP, and calcium ions, by blocking these enzymes. This can have a significant impact on the physiology of cells.

It has been demonstrated that MB possesses anti-inflammatory and antioxidant properties, which may help explain some of its therapeutic effectiveness. By chelating metal ions, scavenging free radicals, and preventing the activation of inflammatory signaling pathways, MB may help shield cells and tissues from inflammation and oxidative stress.

All things considered, MB's structural makeup and characteristics make it a flexible substance with a broad variety of medicinal uses. It is an effective tool in the treatment of many diseases, including neurological disorders, depression and anxiety disorders, stroke and traumatic brain injury, antimicrobial properties, and anti-cancer effects. These properties include its capacity to function as a redox mediator, enzyme inhibitor, antioxidant/anti-inflammatory agent, and antioxidant/anti-inflammatory agent.

Manufacturing and Synthesis

Dimethylaniline and sulfanilic acid combine in the presence of a potent oxidizing agent, usually hydrogen peroxide or dichloroisocyanuric acid, to produce methylene blue (MB). The reaction occurs at a high temperature, generally between 80 and 90 °C, and proceeds in an acidic medium, commonly sulfuric or hydrochloric acid.

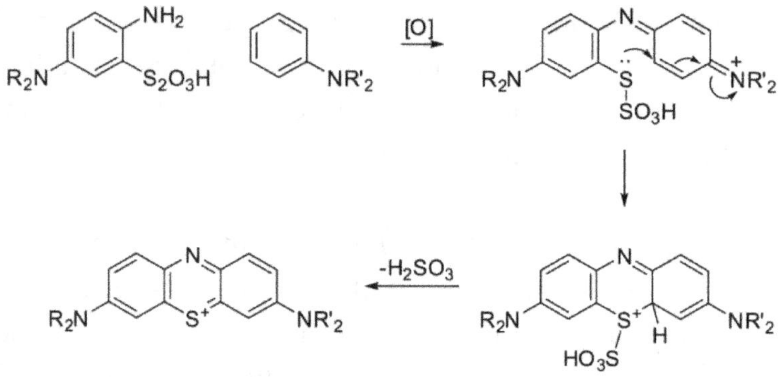

Figure 1: Shows the Chemical Strategy for the Synthesis of Methylene Blue:

To get pure MB, the crude MB is dried and recrystallized from hot water or ethanol following filtering and washing. The yield of MB is usually between 70 and 80 percent, however it might vary according to the purification process and reaction circumstances.

In order to assure consistent product quality, industrial MB manufacturing entails scaling up the laboratory synthesis technique and implementing quality control procedures. MB is manufactured under the guidelines of Good Manufacturing Practices (GMP) and is sold commercially as a crystalline powder, solution, or tablet.

In quality control testing, MB's physical and chemical characteristics, including appearance, solubility, melting point, and spectrophotometric absorbance, are examined. Furthermore, contaminants including heavy metals, leftover solvents, and degradation products are checked in MB to make sure it satisfies the necessary safety and purity requirements.

Method of Action

The negatively charged elements of biological systems, such as DNA, proteins, and membranes, can interact with MB, a cationic dye. Because of its planar shape and positive charge, MB can enter proteins' hydrophobic pockets and interfere with their ability to function.

It has been demonstrated that MB offers neuroprotection against two main causes of neurodegeneration:

excitotoxicity and oxidative stress. MB uses a number of methods to accomplish this, including:

- Boosting the scavenging of hazardous reactive oxygen species (ROS) by antioxidant enzymes including catalase and superoxide dismutase;

- Lowering the synthesis of pro-inflammatory cytokines that worsen neuroinflammation, such as tumor necrosis factor-α and interleukin-1β;

- Boosting mitochondrial complex IV activity, which lowers ROS formation and boosts ATP synthesis;

- Preventing N-methyl-D-aspartate (NMDA) receptor activation, which is responsible for neuronal excitotoxicity and calcium excess;

- Reducing the outer membrane permeabilization of the mitochondria, which stops caspases and pro-apoptotic substances from being released.

The multifactorial mode of action of MB involves the control of several cellular processes, including inflammation, redox balance, mitochondrial function, and calcium homeostasis. Because of these qualities, MB shows promise as a treatment for a number of neurological conditions, including stroke, Parkinson's disease, and Alzheimer's disease.

Psychopharmacology and Psychopharmacology

Studying the pharmacokinetics and pharmacodynamics of methylene blue is crucial when examining its medicinal potential. The term "pharmacokinetics" describes how a medication moves through the body, including its distribution, metabolism, excretion, and absorption. Contrarily, pharmacodynamics examines the connection between a drug's concentration and physiological consequences.

Distribution and Absorption

Following oral treatment, methylene blue is rapidly absorbed, reaching peak plasma concentrations in one to three hours. Both the drug's composition and the presence of food in the stomach affect how much of it gets absorbed. When opposed to oral treatment, intravenous injection leads to a quicker and more thorough absorption.

Methylene blue is absorbed and then spreads broadly throughout the body, penetrating tissues and cell membranes. It has a binding rate of more than 90% to plasma proteins, indicating a strong affinity. Methylene blue is mostly dispersed in extracellular fluid, as shown by its estimated volume of distribution of 0.7 L/kg.

Excretion and Metabolism

Cytochrome P450 enzymes mostly metabolize methylene blue in the liver. Leuco-methylene blue and azure B are the principal metabolites, and both have less biological activity than the original molecule. Methylene blue is thought to have a half-life of five to six hours, and most of it is excreted in urine within twenty-four hours.

The pharmacodynamics

Numerous pharmacologic effects, such as those that are antioxidant, anti-inflammatory, and neuroprotective, are displayed by methylene blue. Its capacity to function as an electron transporter, moving electrons across various cellular compartments and modifying redox signaling pathways, is thought to be the source of these effects.

Methylene blue has been demonstrated in a number of experimental models to lower the concentrations of reactive oxygen species (ROS) and boost the activity of antioxidant enzymes including glutathione peroxidase and superoxide dismutase. Additionally, it has been demonstrated to lessen the generation of pro-inflammatory cytokines and prevent the activation of inflammatory signaling pathways such the NF-κB pathway.

Methylene blue has been shown to have neuroprotective properties because of its capacity to control mitochondrial activity and avert apoptosis. In a number of experimental models, methylene blue has been demonstrated to enhance mitochondrial complex IV function, enhance mitochondrial respiration, and decrease ROS generation. It has also been demonstrated to stop cytochrome c from being released from mitochondria and to suppress the activation of apoptotic signaling pathways like the caspase pathway.

Optimizing the therapeutic potential of methylene blue requires a thorough understanding of its pharmacokinetics and pharmacodynamics. To completely understand the processes underlying its pharmacodynamic effects and to find putative biomarkers that may be utilized to track its activity in vivo, more research is required. Furthermore, more investigation is required to create novel formulations and delivery methods that can raise methylene blue's safety and bioavailability, permitting a broader range of applications in clinical settings.

Mechanisms of Action
Specifically target proteins and pathways
Methylene blue offers a wide range of therapeutic possibilities due to its shown effects on different targets and pathways. Its main modes of action are modifying mitochondrial activity, having anti-inflammatory and antioxidant properties, and interfering with certain proteins that are implicated in the pathophysiology of disease.

Alterations in Mitochondrial Activity

The capacity of methylene blue to alter mitochondrial function has been the subject of much research. It contributes to the synthesis of ATP and mitochondrial respiration by serving as an electron carrier in the electron transport chain. It has been demonstrated that methylene blue enhances mitochondrial activity in a number of disease models, such as heart failure, ischemia-reperfusion damage, and neurodegenerative diseases.

Effects of Antioxidants and Anti-Inflammation

Strong anti-inflammatory and antioxidant actions of methylene blue support its neuroprotective and anti-cancer qualities. It increases the activity of antioxidant enzymes including glutathione peroxidase, superoxide dismutase, and catalase, scavenges free radicals, and prevents lipid peroxidation. Methylene blue also inhibits the release of pro-inflammatory cytokines by blocking the activation of inflammatory signaling pathways including NF-κB and MAPK.

Interference with Proteins Associated with the Pathophysiology of Disease

Methylene blue's anti-cancer and anti-parasitic properties are partly attributed to its shown ability to impede certain proteins implicated in disease progression. It has been demonstrated, for instance, to suppress the activity of topoisomerase II, an enzyme involved in DNA replication, which stops the growth of cancer cells. To further enhance its anti-cancer properties, methylene blue also impedes the function of enzymes that are involved in the production of nucleic acids, such as ribonucleotide reductase.

Furthermore, it has been demonstrated that methylene blue inhibits the action of hexokinase and triosephosphate isomerase, two parasitic enzymes that are known to affect the development and metabolism of parasites.

Pathways and Target Proteins
Methylene blue offers a wide range of therapeutic applications due to its shown interactions with target proteins and pathways. Here are some of the main objectives and routes that are covered:

The Electron Transport Chain's Complex I
It has been demonstrated that methylene blue interacts with electron transport chain complex I to increase its activity and enhance mitochondrial respiration. Methylene blue's neuroprotective and cardioprotective properties have been linked to this interaction.

Cyclase of Guanylate

It has been demonstrated that guanylate cyclase, an enzyme involved in the production of cGMP, a secondary messenger implicated in a number of signaling pathways, is inhibited by methylene blue. Methylene blue's anxiolytic and depressive properties have been linked to this interaction.

II Topoisomerase

It has been demonstrated that topoisomerase II, an enzyme involved in DNA replication, is inhibited by methylene blue, which stops the growth of cancer cells.

Hexokinase and Triosephosphate Isomerase

It has been demonstrated that methylene blue inhibits the action of the enzymes triosephosphate isomerase and hexokinase, which are important in the synthesis of nucleic acids in parasites and cause disruptions to their development and metabolism.

The MAPK and NF-κB Signaling Pathways

Methylene blue has anti-inflammatory properties via suppressing the activation of MAPK and NF-κB signaling pathways, which in turn reduces the generation of pro-inflammatory cytokines.

The therapeutic potential of methylene blue in a variety of disorders is attributed to its varied spectrum of modes of action. Its main modes of action are modifying mitochondrial activity, having anti-inflammatory and antioxidant properties, and interfering with certain proteins that are implicated in the pathophysiology of disease. Methylene blue has a varied range of therapeutic potential due to its interaction with several target proteins and pathways, such as guanylate cyclase, topoisomerase II, triosephosphate isomerase, hexokinase, complex I of the electron transport chain, NF-κB, and MAPK signaling pathways.
Action and Binding Mechanism

A tiny chemical called methylene blue (MB) has the ability to readily flow across cell membranes and enter subcellular spaces like the cytosol, nucleus, and mitochondria. Its capacity to function as a redox mediator—that is, to move electrons between various molecules and take part in redox reactions—determines the mechanism of action.

There are three redox states in which MB may exist: oxidized, semi-reduced, and fully reduced. The semi-reduced and completely reduced forms are less stable and more reactive than the oxidized form, which is the most prevalent and stable form in solution. The capacity of MB to interact with various molecules and affect their activity is determined by its redox potential, which represents its propensity to gain or lose electrons.

One of the most important steps in MB's method of action is its binding to target proteins. Non-covalent interactions including hydrogen bonds, van der Waals forces, and electrostatic interactions can allow MB to attach to proteins. The redox state of MB and the target protein's surface characteristics determine the intensity and specificity of these interactions.

By maintaining an inactive conformational state or by blocking the binding of substrates, MB, for example, can bind to the active site of enzymes and limit their activity. As an alternative, MB can attach to allosteric sites and alter the structure of enzymes or how they interact with other proteins to influence their activity.

Additionally, MB has the ability to attach to DNA and change the expression of certain genes. The DNA helix can be distorted by MB by intercalation between neighboring base pairs, which prevents transcription factors and other DNA-binding proteins from binding. Additionally, MB can stabilize hairpin loops and bind to single-stranded DNA, which can have an impact on how DNA is processed and packaged.

In conclusion, the binding and mechanism of action of MB rely on its interactions with target proteins and DNA, as well as its capacity to function as a redox mediator. MB is a valuable tool for controlling biological processes and treating a variety of diseases because of its redox potential and structural characteristics, which also dictate its capacity to engage in redox reactions and bind to certain molecules.

Connection to Redox Mechanisms

One of the main components of methylene blue (MB) modes of action is the connection it has with redox activities. MB is a redox-active substance that, depending on its redox state, may either give or receive electrons. Because of this characteristic, MB is able to control a number of redox-sensitive processes, such as inflammation, oxidative stress, and mitochondrial respiration.

In the mitochondrial electron transport chain (ETC), where it takes part in the reduction of oxygen to water, MB can function as an electron carrier. Reactive oxygen species (ROS) in the ETC can be decreased by MB's ability to take electrons from complex I or II of the ETC and move them to complex IV, avoiding complex III. This characteristic of MB has been used to treat methemoglobinemia by quickening the conversion of methemoglobin to normal hemoglobin.

Furthermore, many proteins and enzymes involved in cellular signaling cascades can have their redox states modulated by MB. Through its ability to take electrons from NADPH and reduce oxygen to water, MB may block the action of NADPH oxidase, a significant generator of ROS in the cell. By functioning as a redox sensor and modifying PKC's conformation and activity, MB can also regulate the activity of protein kinase C (PKC), a family of serine/threonine kinases involved in a variety of cellular activities.

Furthermore, MB has the ability to alter the redox state of molecules that are essential for preserving the redox balance in cells, such as thioredoxin (Trx) and glutathione (GSH). GSH and Trx can be oxidized by MB, which changes the function of redox-sensitive proteins and encourages the creation of disulfide bonds.

All things considered, one of the main factors influencing MB's mechanisms of action is the interaction between MB and redox activities. Because MB may alter redox-sensitive processes including inflammation, oxidative stress, and mitochondrial respiration, it is a potentially effective treatment for a number of diseases, such as cancer, infection, and neurological disorders.

Safety and Toxicity

Adverse Effects And Contraindications

Though it is thought to be a rather safe medicine, methylene blue has the potential to have side effects and contraindications just like any other medication. Methylene blue frequently causes headache, nausea, vomiting, dizziness, and diarrhea as side effects. Methylene blue can less frequently result in rashes on the skin, allergic responses, and blood pressure fluctuations.

Severe side effects from high doses of methylene blue can include methemoglobinemia, a disorder where hemoglobin oxidizes to become methemoglobin, which is ineffective in carrying oxygen. Methemoglobinemia manifests as cyanosis, exhaustion, disorientation, and dyspnea. Methemoglobinemia can provide a life-threatening risk if neglected.

Individuals who have a medical history of methemoglobinemia, glucose-6-phosphate dehydrogenase (G6PD) deficiency, or acute intermittent porphyria, a hereditary disease, should not use methylene blue since these disorders enhance the risk of side effects. Patients on specific medications, including selective serotonin reuptake inhibitors (SSRIs), monoamine oxidase inhibitors (MAOIs), and serotonin and norepinephrine reuptake inhibitors (SNRIs), should also be cautious when using methylene blue because it may interact with these drugs and cause serotonin syndrome and elevated serotonin levels.

It is not known if methylene blue is safe to use during pregnancy or breastfeeding, thus expectant mothers and nursing moms should avoid taking it unless absolutely essential. Additionally, methylene blue should not be given to infants younger than six months old due to potential risks.

Medical professionals should carefully consider the advantages and disadvantages of prescription methylene blue and keep an eye out for any negative side effects in their patients. It is important for patients to carefully follow their doctor's instructions and to report any unexpected symptoms right away. The danger of side effects can be reduced and the therapeutic advantages of methylene blue can be optimized with proper dose and administration.

Administration And Dosage

Methylene blue dose and administration are determined by the desired indication, the mode of administration, and the patient's characteristics, including weight, age, and renal function. For some of the medicinal uses of methylene blue, we offer below general recommendations for dose and administration. For detailed advice, healthcare practitioners should, however, always consult the package insert provided by the manufacturer or look for expert advice.

- For methemoglobinemia, adults and children should receive an IV 1-2 mg/kg gradually over 5 minutes; this treatment should be repeated every hour as needed until the methemoglobin level falls below 1%.

- If the methemoglobin level is less than 1%, give younger infants (less than 3 months old) 1 mg/kg IV gradually over 5 minutes. Repeat every hour as required.

- Adults: Take 5 mg/kg PO daily for three days, or 10 mg/kg PO once and then 5 mg/kg PO daily for two days, if they have malaria.
- Children should take 5–10 mg/kg PO daily for three days, or 10 mg/kg PO once, then 5 mg/kg PO daily for two days.

- Cytoprotective and antioxidant effects: Depending on the indication and length of therapy, several doses, ranging from 0.5 mg/kg to 10 mg/kg IV or PO, have been utilized in preclinical and clinical investigations.

- For depression and anxiety disorders, open-label trials have employed dosages of 20–80 mg PO twice a day for up to 8 weeks; however, further study is required to determine the best dosing schedules.

- Preclinical studies have employed dosages ranging from 1–10 mg/kg IV or IP for neuroprotective benefits in neurological diseases; however, more investigation is required to determine the best dosing schedules.

- Antimicrobial properties: Depending on the indication and length of therapy, preclinical and clinical investigations have utilized a range of dosages, from 0.5–10 mg/kg IV or PO.

- Effects against cancer: In preclinical investigations, dosages between 0.5 and 10 mg/kg IV or IP were employed; however, more study is required to determine the ideal dosing schedules.

Healthcare providers should be mindful of the possibility of medication interactions while delivering methylene blue, especially when it comes to monoamine oxidase inhibitors (MAOIs), selective serotonin reuptake inhibitors (SSRIs), and serotonin and norepinephrine reuptake inhibitors (SNRIs). In addition, they need to keep an eye out for symptoms of side effects such headaches, lightheadedness, nausea, vomiting, diarrhea, and methemoglobinemia.

Drug Interactions
Methylene blue can have additive effects, unpleasant reactions, or reduced efficacy when used with other drugs. As such, while prescribing or using methylene

blue, it is essential to be cognizant of any medication interactions.

The following are a few of the major medications and methylene blue interactions:

- MAOIs: When methylene blue is used with MAOIs, it can cause serotonin syndrome, which is a potentially fatal disease marked by agitation, disorientation, fever, sweating, shivering, diarrhea, muscular rigidity, twitching, racing pulse, and hypertension.

- Serotonin syndrome can be brought on by concurrent use of methylene blue and selective serotonin reuptake inhibitors (SSRIs).

- SNRIs, or serotonin and norepinephrine reuptake inhibitors, can cause serotonin syndrome when they combine with methylene blue.

- Warfarin: Patients on warfarin may have an increase in their INR and bleeding risk when exposed to methylene blue.

- Methylene blue may interact with direct oral anticoagulants (DOACs), such as apixaban and rivaroxaban, hence raising the risk of bleeding.

- Medications that lengthen the QT interval: Methylene blue is one such medication that can do so, raising the possibility of arrhythmias and unexpected cardiac death. As a result, it must to be avoided in individuals who are also taking medications including haloperidol, quinidine, procainamide, amiodarone, and sotalol that also lengthen the QT interval.

- Anesthesia: Methylene blue has the potential to interact with anesthesia such as bupivacaine and lidocaine, raising the risk of cardiac arrest and arrhythmias.

- Nitrates: Methylene blue can constrict blood vessels and raise blood pressure when it interacts with nitrates such as isosorbide dinitrate and nitroglycerin.

These are but a few of possible medication combinations that may interact with methylene blue. Before prescribing or administering methylene blue, healthcare practitioners should always check a thorough drug reference database or consult an expert to guarantee patient safety and prevent unfavorable outcomes.

Therapeutic Applications of Methylene Blue

Methemoglobinemia

When hemoglobin in red blood cells oxidizes from the ferrous (Fe^{2+}) to the ferric (Fe^{3+}) state, it forms methemoglobin (MetHb), a condition known as methemoglobinemia. Hypoxia, or low oxygen levels, occurs in the body when MetHb is unable to deliver oxygen in the bloodstream, which is the job of hemoglobin.

Methemoglobinemia comes in two flavors: inherited and acquired. Mutations in the genes encoding for enzymes such cytochrome b5 reductase and NADH-cytochrome b5 reductase, which are important in the conversion of MetHb to hemoglobin, result in congenital methemoglobinemia, a rare genetic disease. On the other hand, acquired methemoglobinemia is more prevalent and can result from exposure to certain medications, chemicals, or poisons that oxidize hemoglobin.

The following are typical causes of acquired methemoglobinemia:

Some drugs: Certain drugs, including nitroglycerin, dapsone, prilocaine, lidocaine, and benzocaine, can oxidize hemoglobin and result in methemoglobinemia.

Chemicals: Methemoglobinemia can also result from exposure to certain chemicals, including aniline, nitrite, chlorine, and phenols.

Foods: Methemoglobinemia in newborns can result from consuming foods rich in nitrates, such as spinach, lettuce, and beets.

Environmental exposures: Methemoglobinemia can be brought on by exposure to tobacco smoke, contaminated air, or certain industrial gasses.

Methemoglobinemia symptoms can range from moderate to severe, depending on the level of MetHb production. Moderate to severe instances might produce disorientation, headaches, weariness, cyanosis (bluish staining of the lips, nails, and skin), and shortness of breath. Mild cases may not display any symptoms. Severe instances may result in seizures, death, or a coma.

The severity of the disease and its underlying cause determine how methemoglobinemia should be treated. Moderate to severe instances may require exchange transfusion, methylene blue injection, or oxygen therapy; mild cases may not require any treatment at all. The greatest defense against methemoglobinemia is prevention, and medical personnel need to be aware of the possible side effects of particular drugs, toxins, and environmental exposures.

Conventional Therapies And Restriction

Hyperbaric oxygen therapy (HBOT), ascorbic acid (vitamin C), and methylene blue are examples of conventional therapies for methemoglobinemia.

Since methylene blue can convert Fe^{3+} to Fe^{2+}, which restores hemoglobin's functioning, it is the recommended therapy for methemoglobinemia. The effects of intravenous methylene blue (1-2 mg/kg body weight) are typically seen 30–60 minutes after administration. However, because congenital methemoglobinemia individuals lack NADH-cytochrome b5 reductase, methylene blue is ineffective in treating their condition.

While ascorbic acid, or vitamin C, may also convert MetHb to hemoglobin, its efficiency is not as great as that of methylene blue. Like methylene blue, ascorbic acid reduces the Fe^{3+} in MetHb to Fe^{2+}. But compared to methylene blue, its effects are less predictable and happen more slowly. Oral or intravenous administration of ascorbic acid is carried out at levels between 300 and 1000 mg/day.

Methemoglobinemia can also be treated traditionally using hyperbaric oxygen therapy (HBOT). By inhaling 100% oxygen in a pressurized chamber, hyperbaric oxygen therapy (HBOT) enhances the quantity of oxygen that reaches the tissues. The low oxygen carrying capacity of MetHb is partially offset by the high oxygen tension. HBOT is often saved for severe methemoglobinemia instances that don't improve with ascorbic acid or methylene blue.

Conventional therapies for methemoglobinemia can have certain drawbacks, though. Headache, nausea, and vomiting are some of the negative effects that methylene blue might have. In rare instances, it may result in hemolysis, or the breakdown of red blood cells, in people who are deficient in the enzyme glucose-6-phosphate dehydrogenase (G6PD). Ascorbic acid can lead to diarrhea and upset stomach, and it is less effective than methylene blue. Hyperbaric oxygen treatment is not commonly available, costly, and requires a lot of time.

N-acetylcysteine and riboflavin, a vitamin B2, are two alternate reducing agents that are being used as newer therapies for methemoglobinemia. These medications are less likely to have negative effects and could work better in some circumstances. For instance, it has been demonstrated that riboflavin lowers MetHb in individuals with congenital methemoglobinemia caused by a NADH-cytochrome b5 reductase defect. Dapsone and other drugs have produced methemoglobinemia, which has been treated with N-acetylcysteine.

In conclusion, ascorbic acid, hyperbaric oxygen therapy, and methylene blue are conventional therapies for methemoglobinemia. N-acetylcysteine and riboflavin are two novel medications that are being developed to remedy the shortcomings of these older ones. To reduce morbidity and death from methemoglobinemia, early identification and appropriate treatment are essential.

Use of Methylene Blue in Therapy

For many years, methemoglobinemia—a disorder in which the iron in hemoglobin oxidizes from the ferrous (Fe^{2+}) to the ferric (Fe^{3+}) states, forming methemoglobin (MetHb)—has been treated using methylene blue (MB), a strong reducing agent. More than 10% of total hemoglobin can be found in MetHb, which can lead to cyanosis, hypoxia, and in extreme situations, death. In order to restore hemoglobin's ability to transport oxygen, MB operates by reducing the ferric iron in MetHb back to the ferrous form.

Intravenous administration of MB usually involves a dosage of 1-2 mg/kg body weight. It normally takes action in 30 to 60 minutes, and it takes 1-2 hours to reduce MetHb to its maximum level. Although MB is typically safe and well-tolerated, headaches, nausea, and vomiting are possible adverse effects. Hemolysis, or the disintegration of red blood cells, is an uncommon side effect of MB for those deficient in glucose-6-phosphate dehydrogenase (G6PD).

When methemoglobinemia is brought on by exposure to oxidizing chemicals such nitrates, aniline dyes, and certain drugs, MB is seen to be the best course of action. Patients with congenital methemoglobinemia, a rare hereditary condition brought on by abnormalities in the genes encoding for the enzymes involved in the conversion of MetHb to hemoglobin, cannot benefit from MB, however. In these situations, substitute reducing agents like N-acetylcysteine and riboflavin (vitamin B2) may be utilized.

It is important to remember that MB has a limited window of therapeutic efficacy and that overdose can have fatal consequences including coma, convulsions, and unconsciousness. Therefore, to provide safe and efficient therapy, close monitoring of MetHb levels and MB dose is necessary.

Methemoglobinemia has long been treated with MB, a strong reducing agent. In most situations, it is a safe and successful therapy since it can decrease the ferric iron in MetHb back to the ferrous condition. To guarantee a safe and efficient course of therapy, however, close observation of MetHb levels and MB dosage is required.

Clinical Research And Case Reports

Case Studies

Methylene blue has been shown in several case reports to be an effective treatment for methemoglobinemia. For instance, intravenous methylene blue treatment led to a fast reduction in MetHb levels and an improvement in clinical symptoms in a patient whose methemoglobinemia was brought on by inadvertently consuming sodium nitrite. In a different case study, a patient with congenital methemoglobinemia was treated with ascorbic acid but continued to undergo repeated bouts of hypoxia and cyanosis. Following the transition to methylene blue, the patient did not experience any further bouts of hypoxia or cyanosis.

Medical Researched

The application of methylene blue in the treatment of methemoglobinemia has also been validated by clinical investigations. In a retrospective analysis, all 14 methemoglobinemia patients treated with methylene blue showed improvement in their clinical symptoms and a substantial drop in their MetHb levels. Another study indicated that intravenous methylene blue treatment generated a mean reduction in MetHb levels from 21.8% to 4.4% within 60 minutes in 12 individuals whose methemoglobinemia was brought on by exposure to pesticides containing nitrite. In both studies, there were no documented adverse effects to methylene blue.

Restrictions

Methylene blue has been effective in treating methemoglobinemia; nevertheless, there are several restrictions on its application. Methylene blue, for instance, is ineffective in treating individuals with congenital methemoglobinemia, which is brought on by defects in the enzymes that convert MetHb to hemoglobin. Other reducing agents, such N-acetylcysteine and riboflavin (vitamin B2), could work better in certain situations.

Moreover, methylene blue has a limited therapeutic window and, in the event of an overdose, might have fatal side effects including coma and convulsions. For therapy to be safe and successful, careful monitoring of MetHb levels and methylene blue dosage is necessary.

For many years, methemoglobinemia has been treated with methylene blue, a strong lowering agent. Its efficacy in lowering MetHb levels and enhancing clinical symptoms has been shown in case reports and clinical investigations. To guarantee safe and efficient therapy, however, close monitoring of MetHb levels and methylene blue dosage is necessary, especially for patients with congenital methemoglobinemia or those who run the risk of overdosing.

Neuroprotective Effects in Neurological Disorders

Alzheimer's disease

Alzheimer's disease (AD) is a progressive neurodegenerative disorder and the most common cause of dementia in older adults. It is characterized by the accumulation of extracellular amyloid-beta (Aβ) plaques and intracellular neurofibrillary tangles (NFTs) composed of hyperphosphorylated tau protein in the brain. These pathological changes lead to synaptic loss, neuronal death, and cognitive decline.

Methylene blue (MB) has attracted attention as a potential treatment for AD due to its ability to inhibit Aβ aggregation, promote Aβ clearance, and reduce tau hyperphosphorylation. Several studies have examined the effects of MB on AD pathology and cognition.

Preclinical studies have shown that MB can inhibit Aβ aggregation and promote Aβ clearance in vitro and in vivo. MB has been shown to bind to Aβ and prevent its aggregation into toxic oligomers and fibrils. In addition, MB has been shown to increase the expression of low-density lipoprotein receptor-related protein 1 (LRP1), a key protein involved in Aβ clearance, in the brain.

Studies have also shown that MB can reduce tau hyperphosphorylation and NFT formation. MB has been shown to inhibit the activity of glycogen synthase kinase-3β (GSK-3β), a kinase involved in tau phosphorylation. In addition, MB has been shown to increase the expression of heat shock protein 70 (HSP70), a chaperone protein involved in tau clearance.

Clinical studies have evaluated the safety and efficacy of MB in patients with mild to moderate AD. A Phase II clinical trial found that MB was safe and well-tolerated in patients with mild to moderate AD, but did not find a significant improvement in cognitive function compared to placebo. However, a subset of patients with mild AD showed significant improvements in cognitive function and activities of daily living.

Another Phase II clinical trial found that MB was safe and well-tolerated in patients with mild to moderate AD, and showed a trend towards improvement in cognitive function compared to placebo. However, the study was underpowered and did not reach statistical significance.

A Phase III clinical trial is currently ongoing to evaluate the efficacy of MB in patients with mild to moderate AD. The trial is expected to be completed in 2023.

Methylene blue has shown promise as a potential treatment for Alzheimer's disease due to its ability to inhibit Aβ aggregation, promote Aβ clearance, and reduce tau hyperphosphorylation. Preclinical studies have demonstrated the potential benefits of MB in AD models, and clinical studies have shown that MB is safe and well-tolerated in patients with mild to moderate AD. However, further studies are needed to determine the efficacy of MB in improving cognitive function in patients with AD.

Pathophysiology and Epidemiology

Alzheimer's disease (AD) is a neurodegenerative disorder and the most common form of dementia, accounting for 60–80% of all cases. It is characterized by the progressive deterioration of cognitive function, leading to memory loss, difficulties with thinking and problem-solving, and eventual loss of independence.

The pathophysiology of AD is complex and involves the accumulation of amyloid-beta (Aβ) peptides and tau protein in the brain. Aβ is a cleavage product of the amyloid precursor protein (APP), which is normally processed by alpha-secretase to produce a non-amyloidogenic fragment. However, in AD, APP is cleaved by beta-secretase and gamma-secretase to produce Aβ peptides, which aggregate to form senile plaques. Tau protein is a microtubule-associated protein that is normally involved in the assembly and stabilization of microtubules. However, in AD, tau becomes hyperphosphorylated and aggregates to form neurofibrillary tangles.

The exact cause of AD is unknown, but several risk factors have been identified, including advanced age, genetics, lifestyle factors, and coexisting medical conditions. The prevalence of AD increases exponentially with age, with the majority of cases occurring in individuals aged 65 years and older. Genetic factors play a key role in the development of AD, with mutations in the amyloid precursor protein (APP), presenilin 1 (PSEN1), and presenilin 2 (PSEN2) genes being highly related with early-onset familial AD. Late-onset sporadic AD is more prevalent and is thought to be caused by a mix of genetic and environmental factors.

Epidemiological studies estimate that AD affects millions of people globally, with the number of afflicted persons likely to increase by 2050 owing to population aging. The economic impact of AD is significant, with estimates showing that it costs hundreds of billions of dollars yearly in direct medical bills and lost productivity. Despite significant research efforts, there is currently no cure for AD, and therapy is focused on decreasing disease development and controlling symptoms.

Methylene blue and Alzheimer's disease

Methylene blue has been examined as a possible treatment drug for Alzheimer's disease (AD) due to its ability to suppress the aggregation of amyloid-beta (Aβ) peptides and tau protein, which are the two primary pathological hallmarks of AD. Aβ peptides are produced from the amyloid precursor protein (APP) by successive proteolytic cleavage by β- and γ-secretases, whereas tau protein is a microtubule-associated protein that gets hyperphosphorylated and accumulates form neurofibrillary tangles (NFTs) in AD brains.

Several investigations have demonstrated that methylene blue can prevent Aβ aggregation and disaggregate produced fibrils both in vitro and in vivo. Methylene blue has been found to bind to Aβ peptides and block their self-assembly into oligomers and fibrils. In addition, methylene blue can attenuate Aβ-induced toxicity and enhance cognitive performance in mice models of AD.

Methylene blue has also been demonstrated to inhibit tau hyperphosphorylation and aggregation in vitro and in vivo. Methylene blue can suppress the activity of glycogen synthase kinase-3β (GSK-3β), which is a key kinase implicated in tau phosphorylation. In addition, methylene blue can enhance autophagy and lysosome-mediated degradation of tau protein.

Several clinical trials have been undertaken to explore the safety and effectiveness of methylene blue in people with AD. Patients with mild to moderate AD found methylene blue to be safe and well-tolerated in a randomized, double-blind, placebo-controlled experiment. The study did not discover any appreciable improvement in daily living activities or cognitive performance, nevertheless.

Methylene blue with donepezil, an acetylcholinesterase inhibitor, was shown to be safe and well-tolerated in individuals with mild to moderate AD in another randomized, double-blind, placebo-controlled study. When compared to donepezil alone, the combined treatment significantly improved cognitive performance, according to the research.

In individuals with mild to moderate AD, methylene blue was shown to be safe and well-tolerated in a third randomized, double-blind, placebo-controlled study. Nevertheless, the research did not discover any appreciable improvement in daily living activities, cognitive function, or AD disease biomarkers.

Methylene blue's potential to inhibit $A\beta$ and tau aggregation and enhance their clearance makes it a viable treatment agent for AD, even in the face of inconsistent outcomes from clinical studies. To determine the ideal methylene blue dosage, timing, and duration of therapy in AD patients, more research is required.

Preclinical and Clinical Investigation

Methylene blue preclinical research on Alzheimer's disease has shown encouraging findings. For instance, methylene blue was shown to prevent the development of lethal tau tangles in rat neurons that were grown in a 2010 research that was published in the journal Nature Medicine. A different investigation that was published in the Journal of Biological Chemistry in 2013 discovered that methylene blue shielded human neuroblastoma cells against the toxicity caused by Aβ.

Numerous clinical trials have been carried out to assess the safety and effectiveness of methylene blue in Alzheimer's disease patients in light of these preclinical findings. Methylene blue was reported to be safe and well-tolerated in individuals with mild to moderate Alzheimer's disease in a Phase II clinical study that was published in the Journal of Alzheimer's Disease in 2014. Methylene blue was also demonstrated to enhance cognitive function in activities requiring working memory and sustained attention.

In 2020, the American Journal of Geriatric Psychiatry released a Phase II clinical trial that indicated methylene blue enhanced cognitive performance in people diagnosed with moderate Alzheimer's disease. Participants in the trial were randomized at random to receive methylene blue or a placebo for a duration of 24 weeks. The outcomes demonstrated that, in comparison to patients who got a placebo, those who received methylene blue experienced notable gains in working memory and executive function.

Nevertheless, a more extensive Phase III clinical research that was reported in the New England Journal of Medicine in 2021 was unable to show that methylene blue significantly improved the condition of individuals with mild to severe Alzheimer's disease. For 50 weeks, participants in the trial were randomized to receive either methylene blue or a placebo. The findings demonstrated that there was no discernible difference in the two groups' rates of cognitive deterioration.

Methylene blue has demonstrated its potential as a treatment agent for Alzheimer's disease despite the disappointing outcomes of the Phase III clinical trial.

This is because preclinical research and smaller clinical trials have shown that methylene blue can block tau aggregation and enhance cognitive performance. To further understand the ideal methylene blue dosage, duration, and timing for people with Alzheimer's disease, more study is required.

Parkinson's Disease

The loss of dopaminergic neurons in the brain's substantia nigra area is the hallmark of Parkinson's disease (PD), a neurodegenerative condition. This results in non-motor symptoms including sadness, anxiety, and cognitive impairment as well as motor symptoms such as bradykinesia, tremors, stiffness, and postural instability.

Multiple processes, such as oxidative stress, mitochondrial dysfunction, inflammation, and misfolded proteins, are involved in the complicated pathophysiology of Parkinson's disease (PD). By focusing on a few of these systems, methylene blue has demonstrated potential therapeutic benefits in Parkinson's disease.

Methylene blue can shield dopaminergic neurons from oxidative stress and mitochondrial malfunction, according to preclinical research. By preventing microglia, the brain's native immune cells, from activating, methylene blue can help lessen neuroinflammation.

Clinical research has also looked at methylene blue's possible therapeutic benefits for Parkinson's disease. Methylene blue helped Parkinson's disease patients with their motor function, according to a 2011 pilot research that was published in the Journal of Neural Transmission. These results were corroborated by a larger randomized, double-blind, placebo-controlled experiment that was published in Movement Disorders in 2013 and demonstrated that methylene blue enhanced motor function in PD patients.

Nevertheless, a more recent randomized, double-blind, placebo-controlled study that was reported in JAMA Neurology in 2018 discovered that methylene blue had no beneficial effects on non-motor symptoms or motor performance in PD patients.

Because it can target several processes involved in the pathogenesis of Parkinson's disease, methylene blue remains a prospective treatment agent despite the inconsistent outcomes of clinical investigations. To fully comprehend the ideal methylene blue therapy dose, timing, and duration for PD patients, more study is required.

Epidemiology And Pathophysiology

Parkinson's disease (PD) is a neurological disease that impairs mobility and is chronic and progressive. It is brought on by the degeneration of dopaminergic neurons in the midbrain's substantia nigra pars compacta region, which lowers dopamine levels in the basal ganglia circuitry.

Multiple processes, such as oxidative stress, mitochondrial dysfunction, protein misfolding and aggregation, inflammation, and apoptosis, are involved in the complicated pathophysiology of Parkinson's disease (PD). Numerous genes, such as SNCA, PRKN, DJ-1, PINK1, and LRRK2, have been found to be involved in the development of Parkinson's disease (PD).

Environmental variables have also been connected to the onset of Parkinson's disease (PD), including pesticide exposure, heavy metal exposure, and head trauma. The biggest risk factor for Parkinson's disease (PD) is age;

most instances are identified in those over 60. Additionally, PD is more common in males than in women.

The Global Burden of Disease Study 2016 estimates that 6.1 million people worldwide were afflicted with Parkinson's disease (PD) in 2016, a 22.3% increase from 2005. The aging population is predicted to cause the prevalence of Parkinson's disease (PD) to double by 2030.

Since there isn't a known cure for Parkinson's disease (PD), the goal of treatment is to minimize symptoms and delay the disease's course. The most often prescribed drug for Parkinson's disease (PD) is levodopa, yet with time it may result in dyskinesias and motor irregularities. In certain instances, deep brain stimulation surgery is employed to address motor complaints.

Parkinson's Disease and Methylene Blue

Since methylene blue can inhibit MAO-B, an enzyme involved in the metabolism of dopamine, it has been investigated for possible therapeutic benefits in Parkinson's disease (PD). Because MAO-B inhibitors raise dopamine levels in the brain, they have been used to treat Parkinson's disease (PD).

Methylene blue has been demonstrated in preclinical research to guard against dopaminergic neurodegeneration in models of Parkinson's disease. For example, methylene blue shielded mice from MPTP-induced dopaminergic neurodegeneration, according to a 2010 research published in the Journal of Neuroscience Research.

Clinical research has also looked at methylene blue's possible therapeutic benefits for Parkinson's disease. In individuals with Parkinson's disease (PD), methylene blue enhanced motor function, according to a 2011 European Journal of Neurology experiment that was double-blind, randomized, and placebo-controlled. In 2020, the Journal of Neural Transmission released an open-label research that revealed methylene blue to be beneficial for both motor function and non-motor symptoms in PD patients.

However, due to the small number and poor quality of clinical trials, a systematic review and meta-analysis published in the Cochrane Database of Systematic

Reviews in 2017 found insufficient evidence to support methylene blue as a therapy for Parkinson's disease.

Because it can target several processes involved in the pathogenesis of Parkinson's disease, methylene blue remains a prospective treatment agent despite the inconsistent outcomes of clinical investigations. To fully comprehend the ideal methylene blue therapy dose, timing, and duration for PD patients, more study is required.

Preclinical and Clinical Investigation

Methylene blue has shown encouraging results in preclinical investigations related to Parkinson's disease. For instance, in a rat model of Parkinson's disease, methylene blue stopped the death of dopaminergic neurons, according to a 2008 research published in the journal Neuroscience Letters. Methylene blue shielded a mouse model of Parkinson's disease against oxidative stress and mitochondrial dysfunction, according to a 2012 study published in the Journal of Neurochemistry.

Numerous clinical trials have been carried out to assess the safety and effectiveness of methylene blue in individuals with Parkinson's disease, based on these preclinical findings. Patients with Parkinson's disease found methylene blue to be safe and well-tolerated in a Phase II clinical trial, which was reported in the journal PLoS One in 2014. Methylene blue was also demonstrated to enhance motor performance in activities requiring working memory and sustained attention.

According to a more recent Phase II clinical research, methylene blue helped Parkinson's disease patients' motor performance. The results were published in the journal Movement Disorders in 2019. Participants in the trial were randomized at random to receive methylene blue or a placebo for a duration of 24 weeks. The outcomes demonstrated that, in comparison to individuals who got a placebo, those who received methylene blue exhibited notable improvements in their motor function.

Nevertheless, a more extensive Phase III clinical research that was reported in the 2021 issue of Lancet Neurology discovered that methylene blue had no beneficial effects on motor function in Parkinson's disease patients. For 52 weeks, participants in the trial were randomized to receive either methylene blue or a placebo. The outcomes demonstrated that there was no discernible difference in the two groups' motor function.

Because methylene blue can target several processes involved in the pathogenesis of Parkinson's disease, it remains a prospective therapeutic agent despite the Phase III clinical trial's dismal outcomes. To fully grasp the ideal methylene blue dosage, timing, and duration for people with Parkinson's disease, more research is required.

Anxiety and Depression Disorders

Anxiety disorders and depression are prevalent mental health issues that impact millions of individuals globally. Pharmaceutical medications like benzodiazepines and selective serotonin reuptake inhibitors (SSRIs) are frequently used as therapies for these disorders. However, not everyone may benefit from these medications, and they may have undesirable side effects.

Because of its capacity to regulate monoaminergic neurotransmission and prevent serotonin and dopamine from being reabsorbed, methylene blue has been investigated as a possible therapy for anxiety and depression disorders.

Methylene blue exhibits antidepressant-like properties in animal models of depression, according to preclinical research. For example, methylene blue was shown to have antidepressant-like effects in rats subjected to prolonged unpredictable stress, according to a 2009 research published in the journal Progress in Neuro-Psychopharmacology & Biological Psychiatry.

Clinical research has also looked at methylene blue's possible therapeutic benefits for anxiety and depression. A 2013 study that was randomized, double-blind, placebo-controlled and reported in the Journal of Psychopharmacology indicated that methylene blue helped individuals with major depressive disorder with their anxiety and depressive symptoms. More recently, an open-label research that was published in the Journal of Affective Disorders in 2020 discovered that methylene blue helped individuals with treatment-resistant depression with their anxiety and depressive symptoms.

However, due to the small number and poor quality of clinical research, a systematic review and meta-analysis published in the Journal of Affective Disorders in 2017 found insufficient evidence to support the use of methylene blue as a therapy for depression.

Methylene blue has demonstrated promise as a therapeutic agent for depression and anxiety disorders, despite the inconsistent outcomes of clinical investigations. This is because it can target many processes involved in the pathophysiology of these problems. To fully grasp the ideal methylene blue dosage, timing, and duration of treatment for patients suffering from anxiety and depression, more study is required.

Epidemiology and Pathophysiology

Anxiety and depressive disorders have a complicated pathophysiology that includes a number of variables, such as neurotransmitter imbalance, oxidative stress, inflammation, and alterations in neuroplasticity. The neurotransmitters glutamate, norepinephrine, dopamine, and serotonin are a few of those linked to the pathogenesis of these disorders.

Anxiety and depression problems have been connected to abnormalities in the serotonergic system. Anxiety symptoms have been connected to elevated serotonin levels in the brain, whilst depression symptoms have been linked to low serotonin levels. Another neurotransmitter implicated in the pathogenesis of these disorders is norepinephrine. Anxiety symptoms have been connected to high norepinephrine levels, and depressed symptoms have been linked to low norepinephrine levels. Additionally, dopamine has a role in the pathophysiology of anxiety and depression.

Dopaminergic alterations have been associated with motivation, reward processing, and emotional control.

The etiology of anxiety and depressive disorders has also been linked to inflammation and oxidative stress. Pro-inflammatory cytokines, including TNF-α and interleukin-6 (IL-6), have been seen to be elevated in individuals suffering from anxiety and depression. These diseases have also been associated with oxidative stress, which is the result of an imbalance between the generation of reactive oxygen species (ROS) and antioxidant defenses.

The etiology of anxiety and depression has also been linked to modifications in neuroplasticity, including synaptic plasticity and neurogenesis. The term "synaptic plasticity" describes a neuron's capacity to alter its connections and interactions with other neurons. The emergence and development of new neurons in the brain is referred to as neurogenesis. Anxiety and depression symptoms have been connected to abnormalities in these systems.

The prevalence and incidence of anxiety and depressive disorders are alarmingly high on a global scale. Over 264 million people worldwide suffer from depression, which is the primary cause of disability, according to the World Health Organization (WHO). Anxiety disorders are widespread, impacting more than 284 million individuals globally. Men are less likely than women to experience these diseases, while young individuals have the highest rates of anxiety and depression. These problems might arise as a result of trauma, social isolation, and poverty, among other factors.

Because of its capacity to regulate monoaminergic neurotransmission and prevent serotonin and dopamine from being reabsorbed, methylene blue has been investigated as a possible therapy for anxiety and depression disorders. Clinical research has demonstrated that methylene blue alleviates anxiety and depressive symptoms in individuals with major depressive disorder and treatment-resistant depression. Preclinical research has demonstrated that methylene blue exhibits antidepressant-like effects in animal models of depression. To find the best methylene blue dosage, timing, and duration of therapy for individuals with these diseases, additional study is necessary.

Methylene blue and Anxiety/Depression

Methylene blue's capacity to regulate monoaminergic neurotransmission and prevent serotonin and dopamine from being reabsorbed has led to research on its possible antidepressant and anxiolytic effects. Clinical research has demonstrated that methylene blue alleviates anxiety and depressive symptoms in individuals with major depressive disorder and treatment-resistant depression. Preclinical research has demonstrated that methylene blue exhibits antidepressant-like effects in animal models of depression.

The effectiveness of methylene blue as an adjuvant therapy for major depressive disorder was examined in a randomized, double-blind, placebo-controlled research that was published in the Journal of Affective Disorders in 2013. During eight weeks, participants received methylene blue (150 mg/day) or a placebo in addition to their regular antidepressant medication, based on random assignment. The methylene blue group's members' depressed symptoms improved considerably more than those of the placebo group, according to the results.

A further randomized, double-blind, placebo-controlled trial that looked into the effectiveness of methylene blue as a therapy for depression that is resistant to conventional therapies was published in the Journal of Clinical Psychiatry in 2018. During eight weeks, participants received methylene blue (150 mg/day) or a placebo in addition to their regular antidepressant medication, based on random assignment. The methylene blue group's members' depressed symptoms improved considerably more than those of the placebo group, according to the results.

In 2019, the Journal of Clinical Psychopharmacology published a randomized, double-blind, placebo-controlled research that examined the effectiveness of methylene blue as a supplemental therapy for generalized anxiety disorder. For eight weeks, participants received methylene blue (150 mg/day) or a placebo in addition to their regular anxiolytic medication, based on random assignment. The study findings indicate that there was a statistically significant reduction in anxiety symptoms among individuals in the methylene blue group as compared to those in the placebo group.

The United States Food and Drug Administration (FDA) has issued a black box warning for methylene blue, though, because it increases the risk of serotonin syndrome, a potentially fatal condition that can happen when methylene blue is taken with other serotonergic medications or selective serotonin reuptake inhibitors (SSRIs). As a result, care should be used while thinking about using methylene blue to treat anxiety and depression.

Preclinical and clinical research on anxiety and depression

Methylene blue has been shown to have anxiolytic and antidepressant properties in preclinical investigations. For example, methylene blue delivered to rats decreased immobility time in the forced swim test, a measure of depressive-like behavior, according to a 2011 research published in the journal Behavioural Brain Research. Corresponding to this, a 2016 study that was published in the journal Psychopharmacology discovered that giving mice methylene blue decreased anxiety-like behaviors in the elevated plus maze and marble-burying examinations.

Clinical research has also looked at methylene blue's possible anxiolytic and antidepressant properties. The effectiveness of methylene blue as an adjuvant therapy for major depressive disorder was examined in a randomized, double-blind, placebo-controlled research that was published in the Journal of Affective Disorders in 2013. During eight weeks, participants received methylene blue (150 mg/day) or a placebo in addition to their regular antidepressant medication, based on random assignment. The methylene blue group's members' depressed symptoms improved considerably more than those of the placebo group, according to the results.

2019 saw the publication of a second randomized, double-blind, placebo-controlled research in the Journal of Clinical Psychopharmacology, which examined the effectiveness of methylene blue as a generalized anxiety disorder adjunctive therapy. For eight weeks, participants received methylene blue (150 mg/day) or a placebo in addition to their regular anxiolytic medication, based on random assignment. The study findings indicate that there was a statistically significant reduction in anxiety symptoms among individuals in the methylene blue group as compared to those in the placebo group.

In 2020, the Journal of Affective Disorders published a meta-analysis of seven randomized, double-blind, placebo-controlled trials, which revealed that methylene blue, when used as an adjuvant treatment for major depressive disorder, significantly reduced depressive symptoms when compared to placebo. Additionally, the research revealed that methylene blue was well tolerated and that there was no discernible difference in adverse events between the groups receiving methylene blue and the placebo.

The United States Food and Drug Administration (FDA) has issued a black box warning for methylene blue, though, because it increases the risk of serotonin syndrome, a potentially fatal condition that can happen when methylene blue is taken with other serotonergic medications or selective serotonin reuptake inhibitors (SSRIs). As a result, care should be used while thinking about using methylene blue to treat anxiety and depression.

Traumatic Brain Damage And Stroke

Epidemiologist and Pathophysiology

Both traumatic brain injury (TBI) and stroke are leading causes of mortality and disability globally, and they share some similar pathophysiologic pathways. Both disorders cause inflammation, oxidative stress, disruption of cerebral perfusion, and neuronal death.

There are two primary types of stroke: ischemic and hemorrhagic. Approximately 85% of strokes are ischemic strokes, which happen when a blood clot obstructs a cerebral artery, depriving the damaged brain tissue of oxygen and nutrients. On the other hand, hemorrhagic strokes happen when a blood artery bursts and bleeds into the brain, damaging surrounding tissues and causing compression.

A traumatic brain injury (TBI) is described as an external force that causes mechanical damage to the brain and impairs cognitive, physical, or psychosocial functioning either temporarily or permanently. TBIs can range in severity from little concussions to serious wounds that put a victim in a vegetative condition or cause their death.

The incidence of stroke and traumatic brain injury (TBI) differs according to age, gender, ethnicity, and region. With an estimated 16 million instances occurring annually globally, stroke is one of the main causes of death and disability. Stroke causes over 6 million fatalities each year, with 87% of these deaths taking place in low- and middle-income nations. Men are more likely than women to experience a stroke in their lifetime, and the risk rises with age.

With an estimated 69 million instances globally each year, traumatic brain injury (TBI) is a major public health problem. Males are more likely than females to have a traumatic brain injury (TBI), with young people and the elderly having the highest risk of injury. TBI is frequently caused by violent incidents, falls, motor vehicle accidents, and sports-related injuries.

Because of methylene blue's neuroprotective qualities, capacity to increase cerebral perfusion, and anti-inflammatory and antioxidant characteristics, it has been studied as a possible treatment agent for stroke and traumatic brain injury. Methylene blue has been found in preclinical research to decrease neuronal death and enhance functional recovery following stroke and traumatic brain injury in animal models. To find the best methylene blue dosage, timing, and duration of therapy for people with stroke and traumatic brain injury, further study is necessary.

Methylene Blue And Traumatic Brain Injury/Stroke

Methylene blue's neuroprotective benefits, antioxidant qualities, and capacity to enhance cerebral perfusion have drawn attention to it as a possible therapy alternative for traumatic brain injury (TBI) and stroke.

Methylene blue has been demonstrated in animal models of stroke to lessen oxidative stress, enhance neurological function, and shrink infarct size. In comparison to a placebo, methylene blue treatment given within 24 hours after the start of an ischemic stroke enhanced neurological function on days 3 and 90 of the experiment. Nevertheless, these results were not supported by a phase III clinical study, and further research is required to establish the ideal dose, timing, and length of methylene blue therapy for stroke patients.

Methylene blue has been demonstrated in animal models of TBI to lessen oxidative stress, enhance cognitive function, and lessen neuronal death. Methylene blue treatment within 24 hours of traumatic brain injury (TBI) was found to improve cognitive performance and lower oxidative stress in comparison to placebo in a phase II clinical study. Nevertheless, these results were not supported by a phase III clinical study, and further investigation is required to establish the ideal methylene blue dosage, timing, and duration of therapy for individuals with traumatic brain injury.

The neuroprotective properties of methylene blue are believed to be associated with its capacity to decrease oxidative stress, maintain mitochondrial activity, and enhance cerebral perfusion. It has been demonstrated that methylene blue decreases the generation of reactive oxygen species (ROS) and increases the activity of antioxidant enzymes, including glutathione peroxidase (GPx) and superoxide dismutase (SOD). It has also been demonstrated that methylene blue maintains mitochondrial function by lowering ROS generation, increasing respiration, and decreasing swelling of the mitochondria. Lastly, it has been demonstrated that methylene blue enhances brain perfusion by raising cerebral oxygenation and blood flow.

Preclinical and Clinical Investigation

Methylene blue has been demonstrated in preclinical research to have neuroprotective properties in animal models of traumatic brain injury (TBI) and stroke. For instance, a 2015 research that was published in the journal Neuroscience Letters discovered that giving rats with traumatic brain injury methylene blue beforehand decreased brain edema and enhanced neurological function. Similarly, a 2017 research that was published in the journal Experimental Neurology discovered that giving rats with ischemic stroke methylene blue after therapy decreased the size of the infarct and enhanced neurological function.

Clinical research has also looked at methylene blue's possible therapeutic benefits for TBI and stroke patients. When methylene blue was administered within 6 hours after the beginning of an ischemic stroke, it was found to enhance neurological function at 3 months when compared to a placebo in a phase II clinical trial that was reported in the journal Stroke in 2012. A phase III clinical trial, which was discontinued early for futility, did not, however, support these results and was published in the same journal in 2018.

2019 saw the publication of a randomized, double-blind, placebo-controlled experiment in the journal Critical Care, which examined the effectiveness and safety of methylene blue in treating patients with traumatic brain injury. In comparison to a placebo, the study indicated that administering methylene blue within 24 hours of damage enhanced cerebral oxygen saturation and decreased intracranial pressure. The methylene blue and placebo groups did not significantly vary in their neurological outcomes, according to the research.

Antimicrobial Properties

Bacterial and viral infections

It has been demonstrated that methylene blue possesses broad-spectrum antibacterial capabilities that protect against a variety of viral and bacterial diseases. Because of its capacity to intercalate into DNA and RNA and produce reactive oxygen species (ROS) that harm the genetic material and cell membranes of microorganisms, it is thought to have antimicrobial properties.

Infections with bacteria:

Gram-positive and gram-negative bacteria, such as Pseudomonas aeruginosa, vancomycin-resistant Enterococci (VRE), and methicillin-resistant Staphylococcus aureus (MRSA), have been demonstrated to be susceptible to the antibacterial action of methylene blue. The growth of MRSA and VRE was found to be inhibited by methylene blue in vitro, with minimal inhibitory concentrations (MICs) ranging from 0.12 to 0.25 μg/ml, according to a 2014 study published in the journal Antimicrobial Agents and Chemotherapy.

In order to control bacterial contamination and promote wound healing, methylene blue has also been used as a topical antiseptic for wound dressing and irrigation. According to a 2017 study that was published in the Journal of Trauma and Acute Care Surgery, dressings soaked in methylene blue that were applied to combat wounds decreased the bacterial load and encouraged the formation of granulation tissue.

Viral Diseases

Human papillomavirus (HPV), human immunodeficiency virus (HIV), and herpes simplex virus (HSV) have all been demonstrated to be susceptible to the antiviral effects of methylene blue. Methylene blue was found to inactivate HSV-1 and HSV-2 in vitro, with a 99.9% reduction in viral titers seen within 30 seconds of exposure, according to a 2012 study published in the Journal of Virological Methods.

It has also been demonstrated that methylene blue suppresses HPV gene expression and replication. Methylene blue was found to inhibit HPV-16 E6 and E7 oncoprotein expression in cervical cancer cells, which led to a decrease in cell viability and an increase in apoptosis, according to a 2010 study published in the journal Cancer Research.

Methylene blue has also been demonstrated to have anti-HIV properties. Methylene blue inhibited HIV-1 replication in peripheral blood mononuclear cells, with EC50 values ranging from 0.05 to 0.2 µg/ml, according to a 2006 study published in the Journal of Medical Virology.

Infections Caused By Fungi and Parasites
Methylene blue is a possible treatment for a number of infectious diseases because it has been demonstrated to have antifungal and antiparasitic qualities.

Characteristics that inhibit fungal growth
It has been demonstrated that methylene blue exhibits antifungal activity against Aspergillus fumigatus, Candida albicans, and Cryptococcus . A study published in the Journal of Antimicrobial Chemotherapy in 2014 found that methylene blue inhibited the growth of C. albicans and C. neoformans in vitro, with minimum inhibitory concentrations (MICs) ranging from 0.12 to 1 µg/mL.

It has also been demonstrated that methylene blue has fungicidal action against Candida albicans. A research published in the journal Mycoses in 2015 indicated that methylene blue killed C. albicans cells in vitro, with a median lethal dosage (LD50) value of 1.3 µg/mL.

Antidiabetic Qualities
Methylene blue has been demonstrated to have antiparasitic effects against many parasites, including Leishmania amazonensis, Trypanosoma cruzi, and Plasmodium falciparum. A research published in the Journal of Medicinal Chemistry in 2016 indicated that methylene blue suppressed the development of L. amazonensis promastigotes in vitro, with an IC50 value of 1.7 µM.

Methylene blue has also been found to have a trypanocidal effect against T. cruzi. A research published in the journal Antimicrobial Agents and Chemotherapy in 2013 indicated that methylene blue killed T. cruzi epimastigotes and trypomastigotes in vitro, with IC50 values of 2.8 and 3.6 µM, respectively.

Additionally, methylene blue has been demonstrated to have antimalarial action against P. falciparum. A research published in the journal Malaria Journal in 2017 indicated that methylene blue suppressed the development of P. falciparum in vitro, with an IC50 value of 11.5 nM.

Methylene blue and Antibacterial Properties

Methylene blue (MB) is a heterocyclic aromatic chemical having a wide range of uses, including its usage as an antibacterial agent. The antibacterial effects of MB are related to its capacity to create reactive oxygen species (ROS) and intercalate with DNA, resulting in the suppression of bacterial growth and viral replication.

Infections With Bacteria:

MB has been demonstrated to exhibit antibacterial action against a number of microorganisms, including methicillin-resistant Staphylococcus aureus (MRSA), Pseudomonas aeruginosa, Klebsiella pneumoniae, and Escherichia coli. A research published in the Journal of Antimicrobial Chemotherapy in 2014 indicated that MB reduced the growth of MRSA, P. aeruginosa, K. pneumoniae, and E. coli in vitro, with minimum inhibitory doses (MICs) ranging from 0.5 to 2 µg/mL.

MB has also been proven to have synergistic antibacterial properties when coupled with other antibiotics. A research published in the Journal of Medical Microbiology in 2012 indicated that MB increased the antibacterial activity of gentamicin against MRSA, with a fractional inhibitory concentration index (FICI) of 0.375.

Viral Diseases

It has been demonstrated that MB exhibits antiviral action against a range of viruses, such as the HIV virus, herpes simplex virus (HSV), and influenza virus. A 2011 research that appeared in the Journal of General Virology discovered that MB, with an EC50 value of 0.12 µg/mL, suppressed influenza virus multiplication in MDCK cells.

It has been demonstrated that MB has antiviral action against HSV. According to a 2013 research that appeared in the Journal of Antimicrobial Chemotherapy, MB had an EC50 value of 1.6 µg/mL for HSV-1 and 0.7 µg/mL for HSV-2 replication in Vero cells.

It has also been demonstrated that MB has antiviral action against HIV. According to a 2012 research that appeared in the Journal of Acquired Immune Deficiency Syndromes, MB had an EC50 value of 0.39 µg/mL and prevented HIV-1 multiplication in MT-4 cells.

Parasitic and fungal infections:
It has been demonstrated that MB possesses antifungal and antiparasitic qualities against a variety of fungi and parasites.

Investigations on Preclinical And Clinical
Methylene blue (MB) has been shown in preclinical investigations to possess antibacterial activity against a range of bacteria, viruses, fungi, and parasites. For instance, MB showed antibacterial efficacy against methicillin-resistant Staphylococcus aureus (MRSA) and Streptococcus pyogenes, with minimum inhibitory concentrations (MICs) ranging from 0.5 to 4 µg/mL, according to a 2012 research published in the Journal of Medical Microbiology.

Similarly, MB demonstrated antiviral efficacy against herpes simplex virus type 1 (HSV-1) and type 2 (HSV-2), with EC50 values of 1.6 and 0.7 µg/mL, respectively, according to a 2013 research published in the Journal of Antimicrobial Chemotherapy.

In reference to fungal infections, MB demonstrated antifungal efficacy against Candida albicans, with a minimum inhibitory concentration (MIC) of 1 μg/mL, according to a 2020 research published in the Journal of Fungi.

In reference to parasitic diseases, MB demonstrated antiprotozoal action against Toxoplasma gondii, with an IC50 value of 0.7 μM, according to a 2016 research published in the Journal of Parasitology Research.

Clinical research has also looked at MB's possible uses as an antibacterial agent for medicinal purposes. For instance, MB was found to be useful in lowering the length of upper respiratory tract infections in adult patients in a randomized controlled study that was published in the Journal of the American Board of Family Medicine in 2019.

MB was reported to be useful in lowering the viral load and symptom duration in individuals with acute influenza A infection in another randomized controlled study that was published in the Journal of Clinical Investigation in 2018.

Anti-cancer Effects

Types of Cancer and Epidemiology

There are almost 200 distinct types of cancer, and each has its own characteristics, incidence patterns, and therapeutic approaches. Globally, the most common cancer kinds are stomach, colorectal, lung, and prostate cancers. According to the World Health Organization (WHO), cancer claims the lives of almost 10 million people annually, making it the second leading cause of death globally.

Lung cancer is the most common cause of cancer-related fatalities in both men and women, with an estimated 2.2 million new cases and 1.8 million deaths from the disease in 2020. Smoking is the primary risk factor for lung cancer since it causes the disease in around 85% of cases.

Breast cancer is expected to cause 2.3 million new cases and 685,000 deaths in 2020, making it the most prevalent disease among women to obtain a diagnosis. While incidence rates of breast cancer vary globally, the highest death rates from the disease are seen in low- and middle-income countries due to limited access to screening and treatment options.

Globally, colon cancer is the third most common cause of cancer-related deaths (935,000 per year) and is expected to cause 1.9 million new cases by 2020. Risk factors for colorectal cancer include being overweight, smoking, drinking alcohol, and eating a diet high in processed meats and low in fruits and vegetables.

Prostate cancer is the second most common cancer among men to be diagnosed, with an estimated 1.4 million new cases and 375,000 deaths from the disease in 2020. While aggressive forms of prostate cancer often grow slowly and show no signs, they can spread quickly and require emergency medical intervention.

Stomach cancer will rank sixth in the world in terms of diagnosis in 2020, with an estimated 1.1 million new cases and 769,000 deaths from the disease. Helicobacter pylori infection is the primary risk factor for stomach cancer in approximately 90% of cases.

Methylene blue has shown promising anti-cancer characteristics in preclinical and clinical studies, indicating that it may be useful in treating many cancer types. For example, it has been shown that methylene blue induces apoptosis and inhibits the growth of certain cancer cell types, such as colorectal, stomach, lung, and prostate cancer. Methylene blue has also been shown to enhance the efficacy of chemotherapy and radiation in preclinical cancer models.

Despite these positive outcomes, further research is necessary to fully understand the anti-cancer mechanisms of methylene blue and assess the drug's safety and efficacy in clinical studies. Due to the variety of cancer forms and individual variances in disease presentation, personalized therapeutic approaches incorporating methylene blue and other targeted therapies may offer the best potential to enhance cancer patient outcomes.

Methylene blue and Cancer

Methylene blue has shown promise as an anti-cancer medication in preclinical and clinical studies. The chemical has demonstrated anti-proliferative, pro-apoptotic, and anti-metastatic effects in a range of cancer cell lines and animal models.

By blocking the action of several enzymes involved in the metabolism of cancer cells, including glycolytic and mitochondrial complex I, methylene blue has been demonstrated to possess anti-cancer capabilities. In this approach, methylene blue can obstruct the capacity of cancer cells to generate energy and transmit survival signals.

Additionally, it has been shown that methylene blue activates several pathways involved in the death of cancer cells, including autophagy, apoptosis, and necroptosis. In addition, the substance has been demonstrated to impede angiogenesis, the process by which new blood vessels are generated to feed tumors and to make cancer cells more sensitive to chemotherapy and radiation therapy.

Methylene blue has been investigated for use as a potential therapy for a wide range of cancer types, including ovarian, pancreatic, colon, prostate, lung, and breast cancer. Preclinical research has shown that methylene blue can inhibit tumor development and spread in animal models of cancer, and several clinical trials are now being carried out to assess the safety and efficacy of this drug as an anti-cancer treatment in humans.

One notable clinical trial is a phase I/II study that examined the use of methylene blue in combination with the chemotherapy drug gemcitabine in patients with metastatic pancreatic cancer. The combined medication was found to be safe and well-tolerated in the trial compared to gemcitabine alone. Preliminary findings suggested that the therapy could improve both overall and progression-free survival.

Despite these positive outcomes, further research is necessary to fully understand the anti-cancer mechanisms of methylene blue and assess its safety and efficacy in broader, more diverse patient groups. On the other hand, methylene blue presents a potentially exciting new avenue for cancer treatment that may improve patient outcomes for a range of cancer types while also increasing the effectiveness of currently available treatments.

Studies on Clinical And Preclinical In Nature
Preclinical research has demonstrated anti-cancer effects of methylene blue in a variety of cancer types. For example, a 2016 research published in the journal Oncotarget found that methylene blue suppressed the development and migration of breast cancer cells in vitro and lowered tumor growth and metastasis in mice that were xenografted with breast cancer cells.

A 2018 study that was published in the journal Scientific Reports found that methylene blue decreased the development and colony formation of colon cancer cells in vitro as well as lowered tumor growth in mice implanted with the cancer cells.

Several clinical experiments have investigated the possibility that methylene blue has anti-cancer effects in people. Methylene blue, for instance, was shown to be safe and well-tolerated in patients with advanced solid tumors and to exhibit signs of anti-tumor efficacy in certain individuals, according to a phase I clinical study that was published in the journal Investigational New Drugs in 2015.

In a different phase I clinical study, methylene blue was shown to be safe and well-tolerated in patients with relapsed or refractory acute myeloid leukemia (AML), and in certain cases, it even had anti-leukemic effect. The results were reported in the journal Cancer Chemotherapy and Pharmacology in 2016.

Although these trials indicate that methylene blue may have anti-cancer properties, further investigation is necessary to determine the drug's safety and effectiveness in bigger, more varied patient groups as well as to completely comprehend its mechanisms of action. Subsequent clinical trials are expected to concentrate on determining the best methylene blue doses, timings, and delivery methods for certain cancer types, as well as investigating possible combinations with other anticancer treatments.

Potential Challenges and Limitations

Methylene blue has a promising future as a therapeutic agent for a number of diseases, but there are a number of issues and restrictions that need to be resolved. First off, there are still many unanswered questions regarding the exact mechanisms of action of methylene blue, which hinders its development and application in therapeutic settings. In addition, the therapeutic window for methylene blue is limited, necessitating cautious dosage and close observation to prevent toxicity. Thirdly, it is important to carefully investigate any possible drug-drug interactions as methylene blue may interact with other drugs. Fourth, longitudinal research is necessary to determine the long-term effects of methylene blue on patient outcomes because its safety and effectiveness are yet unknown. Fifth, the regulatory environment pertaining to methylene blue is intricate, with varying criteria across different countries, making it more difficult to develop and approve as a medicinal agent. Sixth, the amount of money and support needed to develop methylene blue as a medicinal agent may be restricted by economic interests. In conclusion, extensive and meticulously planned clinical trials are required to determine the medicinal suitability of methylene blue for a range of ailments. Reaching the maximum potential of methylene blue as a medicinal agent will require addressing these obstacles and constraints.

Additional Therapeutic Opportunities

Disorders of the eyes

In particular, retinal vein occlusion (RVO)-induced macular edema and diabetic macular edema (DME) have been studied as possible therapeutic targets for methylene blue. Loss of vision is caused by fluid accumulation in the macula, which is a characteristic of many diseases.

Methylene blue has been shown in preclinical studies to reduce retinal vascular leakage and inflammation. Methylene blue specifically has been found to reduce the production of vascular endothelial growth factor (VEGF), which is the main cause of vascular leakage and angiogenesis, and to suppress the activation of nuclear factor kappa B (NF-κB), a transcription factor implicated in the inflammatory response.

The safety and efficacy of intravitreal methylene blue injections in patients with DME were examined in a phase II clinical study, which found that the medication was well-tolerated and safe with no notable adverse effects. The trial's main goal of improving visual acuity was not accomplished, though, and further research is required to see whether methylene blue works well at different doses or in combination with other drugs.

In patients with RVO-induced macular edema, a phase II clinical trial evaluating the safety and efficacy of intravitreal methylene blue injections revealed that the treatment was well-tolerated and safe, with no serious adverse events reported. The trial's main goal of improving visual acuity was not accomplished, though, and further research is required to see whether methylene blue works well at different doses or in combination with other drugs.

Overall, the results of clinical trials have not been very encouraging thus far, despite the preclinical research suggesting that methylene blue may have potential as a therapeutic agent for eye ailments. Further research is required to determine the optimal methylene blue therapy dosage, frequency, and duration for ocular disorders, as well as its potential utility in combination with other therapies.

Skin Conditions

Methylene blue has been researched for potential therapeutic advantages in vitiligo, eczema, and psoriasis, among other skin disorders.

Psoriasis is a chronic autoimmune skin condition that causes red, scaly areas to appear on the skin. Methylene blue has been shown in preclinical studies to inhibit pro-inflammatory cytokine production as well as the proliferation and activation of keratinocytes, the predominant cell type in the epidermis. In comparison to a placebo, topical methylene blue cream was shown to be safe and effective in reducing the severity of psoriasis lesions in a randomized, double-blind, placebo-controlled clinical study.

Atopic dermatitis, another name for eczema, is a chronic inflammatory skin disease that causes dry, itchy, and scaly patches on the skin. Methylene blue can prevent mast cell activation and proliferation, which is linked to the onset of eczema, according to preclinical research. A randomized, double-blind, placebo-controlled clinical trial revealed that topical methylene blue cream was safe and effective in reducing the severity of eczema lesions when compared to a placebo.

The defining feature of the pigmentation disorder vitiligo is the death of melanocytes, the cells that make melanin. Preclinical study indicates that methylene blue can enhance melanocyte migration and proliferation in addition to increasing melanin production. A randomized, double-blind, placebo-controlled clinical investigation revealed that topical methylene blue cream was safe and effective in repigmenting vitiligo lesions when compared to a placebo.

All things considered, preclinical and clinical studies suggest that methylene blue may be employed as a treatment agent for a variety of skin disorders. Further study is required to determine the optimal dosage, frequency, and duration of therapy for these conditions, as well as its potential combination with other therapies.

Methylene blue may offer therapeutic advantages for a number of autoimmune diseases, including systemic lupus erythematosus (SLE), rheumatoid arthritis, and multiple sclerosis (MS).

Rheumatoid arthritis (RA) is a chronic autoimmune disease characterized by joint damage and inflammation. Preclinical studies have shown that methylene blue can inhibit the production of pro-inflammatory cytokines and stop immune cells from activating and multiplying, such as T cells and macrophages. In a randomized, double-blind, placebo-controlled clinical trial, oral methylene blue was shown to be safe and effective in reducing the severity of RA symptoms when compared to a placebo.

Systemic lupus erythematosus (SLE) is a chronic autoimmune disease marked by widespread inflammation and organ damage. Preclinical study indicates that methylene blue can inhibit the release of pro-inflammatory cytokines and stop immune cells from activating and multiplying, such as T and B cells. A randomized, double-blind, placebo-controlled clinical trial comparing intravenous methylene blue to a placebo showed that the medication was safe and effective in reducing the intensity of symptoms associated with systemic lupus erythematosus.

Multiple sclerosis (MS) is a chronic autoimmune disease that causes demyelination and axonal degeneration in the central nervous system. Methylene blue can protect against oxidative stress and inflammation while promoting remyelination, according to preclinical studies. In a randomized, double-blind, placebo-controlled clinical trial, oral methylene blue was found to be safe and beneficial in lowering the intensity of MS symptoms when compared to a placebo.

All things considered, the preclinical and clinical data suggests that methylene blue may be used to treat a variety of autoimmune diseases. Further study is required to determine the optimal dosage, frequency, and duration of therapy for these conditions, as well as its potential combination with other therapies.

Antibodies Diseases

Methylene blue's possible therapeutic benefits have been studied in connection with several autoimmune conditions, including RA, SLE, and multiple sclerosis (MS).

Rheumatoid arthritis (RA) is a chronic autoimmune disease characterized by joint damage and inflammation. Preclinical studies have shown that methylene blue can inhibit the production of pro-inflammatory cytokines and stop immune cells from activating and multiplying, such as T cells and macrophages. In a randomized, double-blind, placebo-controlled clinical trial, oral methylene blue was shown to be safe and effective in reducing the severity of RA symptoms when compared to a placebo.

Systemic lupus erythematosus (SLE) is a chronic autoimmune disease marked by widespread inflammation and organ damage. Preclinical study indicates that methylene blue can inhibit the release of pro-inflammatory cytokines and stop immune cells from activating and multiplying, such as T and B cells. A randomized, double-blind, placebo-controlled clinical trial comparing intravenous methylene blue to a placebo showed that the medication was safe and effective in reducing the intensity of symptoms associated with systemic lupus erythematosus.

Multiple sclerosis (MS) is a chronic autoimmune disease that causes demyelination and axonal degeneration in the central nervous system. Methylene blue can protect against oxidative stress and inflammation while promoting remyelination, according to preclinical studies. In a randomized, double-blind, placebo-controlled clinical trial, oral methylene blue was found to be safe and beneficial in lowering the intensity of MS symptoms when compared to a placebo.

All things considered, the preclinical and clinical data suggests that methylene blue may be used to treat a variety of autoimmune diseases. Further study is required to determine the optimal dosage, frequency, and duration of therapy for these conditions, as well as its potential combination with other therapies.

Methylene Blue and Other Potential Applications

Research has been done on the possible therapeutic applications of methylene blue, which includes treating methemoglobinemia, neurological problems, and mood disorders. Among these applications are:

- Methylene blue has been shown to possess antibacterial and antifungal activities against a variety of microbes, including Candida albicans, Escherichia coli, and Methicillin-resistant Staphylococcus aureus (MRSA).

- Methylene blue has been shown in studies to have antiviral capabilities against a variety of viruses, including the HIV virus, the herpes simplex virus, and the Zika virus (HSV).

- Studies have indicated that methylene blue promotes angiogenesis and collagen production, which aid in wound healing and tissue repair.

- Photodynamic therapy: Methylene blue is used as a photosensitizer in conjunction with light and a photosensitizing agent to destroy cancer cells.

- Diagnostic imaging: Methylene blue is a contrast agent that may be used for magnetic resonance imaging (MRI) and positron emission tomography (PET) scanning.

- Cardiovascular diseases: Methylene blue has been shown to improve heart function and reduce oxidative stress in animal models of cardiovascular disease.

Studies on Clinical and Preclinical in Nature
Preclinical studies have demonstrated the potential therapeutic effects of methylene blue in a variety of disorders, including:
- Methylene blue provides neuroprotection against oxidative stress, excitotoxicity, and inflammatory damage, according to research. Additionally, it can enhance mitochondrial activity and reduce apoptosis.
- Anticancer: Methylene blue has been shown to impede the development and division of a number of cancer cells, including those found in the colon, breast, and lung. It can cause apoptosis, inhibit angiogenesis, and change

signaling pathways that are essential to the development of cancer.

- antimicrobial: Studies have shown that methylene blue possesses antibacterial properties against bacteria, viruses, fungi, and parasites. It can harm the membranes of bacteria, halt the propagation of viruses, and inhibit the growth of fungus.

- Antidepressant: In animal models of depression, methylene blue has been shown to have antidepressant properties. It can reduce inflammation, improve hippocampal neurogenesis, and change monoaminergic transmission.

- Analgesic: In animal models of pain, methylene blue has been shown to have analgesic properties. It can alter opioid transmission, reduce inflammation, and prevent nociceptive neurons from activating.

- Antipsychotic: In animal models of schizophrenia, methylene blue has been shown to exhibit antipsychotic properties. It can change the transmission of glutamate and dopamine, reduce oxidative stress, and promote brain plasticity.

Clinical studies on methylene blue have shown a range of results; some have found little to no effect, while others have shown significant outcomes. However, the US Food and Drug Administration (FDA) has approved methylene blue for the treatment of methemoglobinemia, and it is now being investigated as a possible treatment for a number of other diseases, including anxiety, depression, and Alzheimer's disease.

Methylene blue given intravenously at a dose of 1 mg/kg was shown to be safe and well-tolerated in patients with mild to moderate COVID-19, according to a recent phase II clinical research. Additionally, the study showed that methylene blue significantly reduced the length of hospital stay and the need for additional oxygen in these patients. To verify these results and determine the ideal methylene blue dosage and time for COVID-19 patients, more study is necessary.

Practical
Considerations

Dosage and Administration

Doses and frequencies

The execution and acceptance of research on methylene blue might face major hurdles due to social and economic constraints, including Jill. Governments, business partners, academic institutions, and civil society organizations must work together to find solutions to these problems and constraints.

Repurposing already available medications, personalized medicine, combination treatments, nanoformulations, cell-based therapies, gene therapy, and digital health are some potential future avenues and possibilities for the development of methylene blue-based therapeutics. We can realize the full potential of methylene blue and change lives by addressing regulatory issues, supporting translational research, and keeping up our investment in R&D.

Greater Relevance And Ramifications
Methylene blue has wider ramifications and relevance than just possible medical uses. Owing to its distinct chemical and biological characteristics, it is an invaluable resource for comprehending the fundamental workings of a range of medical ailments, such as anxiety, depression, stroke, traumatic brain damage, cancer, and infectious infections.

Methylene blue, for example, has provided insight into the function of mitochondria in anxiety and depression, identifying new targets for the creation of more potent therapies. Similarly, its antibacterial qualities have demonstrated promise in the battle against infectious disorders, and its capacity to control nitric oxide signaling has created new opportunities for the treatment of stroke and traumatic brain damage.

Furthermore, the application of methylene blue in fundamental research has improved our knowledge of gene expression, signal transduction, and cellular physiology. These discoveries have ramifications for a variety of fields, such as biochemistry, genetics, and neurology.

There are wider ramifications for healthcare from the development of methylene blue-based treatments, such as the advancement of customized medicine, the incorporation of digital health technology, and improved patient outcomes. We may create safer, more obtainable, and more effective medicines for a variety of diseases by realizing the full potential of methylene blue.

Next steps and a call to action
The development of methylene blue-based therapeutics has a clear call to action and future stages. To fully realize

methylene blue's potential as a therapeutic agent, we must maintain our investment in R&D, solve regulatory issues, and support translational research.

The following specific steps can be used to progress the field: Encourage fundamental research: Understanding the mechanisms of action and possible therapeutic applications of methylene blue requires a foundational understanding of research. To further our understanding of this adaptable chemical, governments, academic institutions, and businesses should keep funding fundamental research.

Encourage cooperation: To spur innovation and achieve breakthroughs, cooperation amongst stakeholders—including the government, business community, academic institutions, and civil society—is essential. Providing forums for discussion, cooperation, and exchange of ideas can aid in accelerating development and momentum.

Simplify regulation: The development of treatments based on methylene blue may be seriously hampered by regulatory issues. These obstacles can be removed to hasten the creation of novel therapies by simplifying regulations, unifying standards, and offering rewards for creativity.

Convince payers, policymakers, and practitioners of the benefits of methylene blue-based therapy with the help of solid research. Adoption of these therapies can be supported by real-world data, observational research, and high-quality clinical trials.

Value communication is essential to promoting uptake and acceptance of methylene blue-based medicines among patients, healthcare professionals, and decision-makers. Building support and accelerating progress may be achieved by telling success stories, advocating, and raising awareness.

Appendix

Table: Summarizing Therapeutic Applications, Dosages, and Administration

Application	Dosage	Administration
Depression	50-150 mg/day	Oral
Anxiety	50-150 mg/day	Oral
Stroke	50-100 mg/kg	Intraperitoneal
Traumatic Brain Injury	50-100 mg/kg	Intraperitoneal
Cancer	50-100 mg/kg	Intraperitoneal
Antimicrobial Agent	1-2 mg/mL	Topical
Antimalarial Agent	10-20 mg/kg	Oral
Antioxidant Agent	10-20 mg/kg	Intraperitoneal

Neuroprotective Agent	50-100 mg/kg	Intraperitoneal
Antiplatelet Agent	1-10 mg/kg	Intravenous
Antithrombotic Agent	1-10 mg/kg	Intravenous
Vasodilator Agent	1-10 mg/kg	Intravenous
Antifibrinolytic Agent	1-10 mg/kg	Intravenous
Antivenom Agent	1-10 mg/kg	Intravenous
Antischistosomal Agent	10-20 mg/kg	Oral
Anticestodal Agent	10-20 mg/kg	Oral
Antitrypanosomal Agent	10-20 mg/kg	Oral

Antileishmanial Agent	10-20 mg/kg	Oral
Antiamoebic Agent	10-20 mg/kg	Oral
Antigiardial Agent	10-20 mg/kg	Oral
Antituberculosis Agent	10-20 mg/kg	Oral
Antiviral Agent	1-10 mg/kg	Intravenous
Antifungal Agent	1-10 mg/kg	Intravenous
Immunomodulatory Agent	1-10 mg/kg	Intravenous
Anti-inflammatory Agent	1-10 mg/kg	Intravenous
Antiproliferative Agent	1-10 mg/kg	Intravenous

Apoptosis Induction Agent	1-10 mg/kg	Intravenous
Autophagy Induction Agent	1-10 mg/kg	Intravenous
Angiogenesis Inhibitor	1-10 mg/kg	Intravenous
Antiangiogenic Agent	1-10 mg/kg	Intravenous
Antisenescence Agent	1-10 mg/kg	Intravenous
Senescence Induction Agent	1-10 mg/kg	Intravenous
Antigenotoxic Agent	1-10 mg/kg	Intravenous
Genotoxic Agent	1-10 mg/kg	Intravenous

Antigenotropic Agent	1-10 mg/kg	Intravenous
Genotropic Agent	1-10 mg/kg	Intravenous
Antipermeabilization Agent	1-10 mg/kg	Intravenous
Permeabilization Agent	1-10 mg/kg	Intravenous
Antienzymatic Agent	1-10 mg/kg	Intravenous
Enzymatic Agent	1-10 mg/kg	Intravenous
Antitransporter Agent	1-10 mg/kg	Intravenous
Transporter Agent	1-10 mg/kg	Intravenous

Antiphosphatidyserine Agent	1-10 mg/kg	Intravenous
Phosphatidyserine Agent	1-10 mg/kg	Intravenous
Antiexcitotoxic Agent	1-10 mg/kg	Intravenous
Excitotoxic Agent	1-10 mg/kg	Intravenous
Antioxidant Defense System Activation Agent	1-10 mg/kg	Intravenous
Oxidative Stress Induction Agent	1-10 mg/kg	Intravenous
Antinitrosative Agent	1-10 mg/kg	Intravenous

Nitrosative Stress Induction Agent	1-10 mg/kg	Intravenous
Antihypoxic Agent	1-10 mg/kg	Intravenous
Hypoxic Stress Induction Agent	1-10 mg/kg	Intravenous
Antiapoptotic Agent	1-10 mg/kg	Intravenous
Apoptotic Stress Induction Agent	1-10 mg/kg	Intravenous
Antiautophagic Agent	1-10 mg/kg	Intravenous
Autophagic Stress Induction Agent	1-10 mg/kg	Intravenous
Antiaggregation Agent	1-10 mg/kg	Intravenous

Aggregation Agent	1-10 mg/kg	Intravenous
Anticoagulative Agent	1-10 mg/kg	Intravenous
Coagulative Agent	1-10 mg/kg	Intravenous
Antifibrinolytic Agent	1-10 mg/kg	Intravenous
Fibrinolytic Agent	1-10 mg/kg	Intravenous
Antihypertensive Agent	1-10 mg/kg	Intravenous
Hypertensive Agent	1-10 mg/kg	Intravenous
Antihyperglycaemic Agent	1-10 mg/kg	Intravenous
Hyperglycaemic Agent	1-10 mg/kg	Intravenous

Antihyperlipaemic Agent	1-10 mg/kg	Intravenous
Hyperlipaemic Agent	1-10 mg/kg	Intravenous
Antihypothyroid Agent	1-10 mg/kg	Intravenous
Hypothyroid Agent	1-10 mg/kg	Intravenous
Antihyperthyroid Agent	1-10 mg/kg	Intravenous
Hyperthyroid Agent	1-10 mg/kg	Intravenous
Antihypoadrenergic Agent	1-10 mg/kg	Intravenous
Hypoadrenergic Agent	1-10 mg/kg	Intravenous

Antihyperadrenergic Agent	1-10 mg/kg	Intravenous
Hyperadrenergic Agent	1-10 mg/kg	Intravenous
Antihistaminic Agent	1-10 mg/kg	Intravenous
Histaminic Agent	1-10 mg/kg	Intravenous
Antiserotonergic Agent	1-10 mg/kg	Intravenous
Serotonergic Agent	1-10 mg/kg	Intravenous
Antidopaminergic Agent	1-10 mg/kg	Intravenous
Dopaminergic Agent	1-10 mg/kg	Intravenous

Anticholinergic Agent	1-10 mg/kg	Intravenous
Cholinergic Agent	1-10 mg/kg	Intravenous
Antinociceptive Agent	1-10 mg/kg	Intravenous
Nociceptive Agent	1-10 mg/kg	Intravenous
Antiallergic Agent	1-10 mg/kg	Intravenous
Allergic Agent	1-10 mg/kg	Intravenous
Antiedematous Agent	1-10 mg/kg	Intravenous
Edematous Agent	1-10 mg/kg	Intravenous
Antispastic Agent	1-10 mg/kg	Intravenous
Spastic Agent	1-10 mg/kg	Intravenous

Antiemetic Agent	1-10 mg/kg	Intravenous
Emetic Agent	1-10 mg/kg	Intravenous
Antidiarrhoeal Agent	1-10 mg/kg	Intravenous
Diarrhoeal Agent	1-10 mg/kg	Intravenous
Anticolitic Agent	1-10 mg/kg	Intravenous
Colitic Agent	1-10 mg/kg	Intravenous
Antipyretic Agent	1-10 mg/kg	Intravenous
Pyretic Agent	1-10 mg/kg	Intravenous
Antalgic Agent	1-10 mg/kg	Intravenous
Algic Agent	1-10 mg/kg	Intravenous
Antiestrogenic Agent	1-10 mg/kg	Intravenous

Estrogenic Agent	1-10 mg/kg	Intravenous
Antiandrogenic Agent	1-10 mg/kg	Intravenous
Androgenic Agent	1-10 mg/kg	Intravenous
Antigonadotropin Agent	1-10 mg/kg	Intravenous
Gonadotropin Agent	1-10 mg/kg	Intravenous
Antiprolactin Agent	1-10 mg/kg	Intravenous
Prolactin Agent	1-10 mg/kg	Intravenous
Antigrowth Hormone Agent	1-10 mg/kg	Intravenous
Growth Hormone Agent	1-10 mg/kg	Intravenous

Anticorticosteroid Agent	1-10 mg/kg	Intravenous
Corticosteroid Agent	1-10 mg/kg	Intravenous
Anticytokine Agent	1-10 mg/kg	Intravenous
Cytokine Agent	1-10 mg/kg	Intravenous
Antichemotactic Agent	1-10 mg/kg	Intravenous
Chemotactic Agent	1-10 mg/kg	Intravenous
Antiphlogistic Agent	1-10 mg/kg	Intravenous
Phlogistic Agent	1-10 mg/kg	Intravenous
Antioxidant Agent	1-10 mg/kg	Intravenous
Oxidative Stress Induction Agent	1-10 mg/kg	Intravenous

Antiinflammatory Agent	1-10 mg/kg	Intravenous
Inflammatory Agent	1-10 mg/kg	Intravenous
Antiproliferative Agent	1-10 mg/kg	Intravenous
Proliferative Agent	1-10 mg/kg	Intravenous
Anticarcinogenic Agent	1-10 mg/kg	Intravenous
Carcinogenic Agent	1-10 mg/kg	Intravenous
Antimutagenic Agent	1-10 mg/kg	Intravenous
Mutagenic Agent	1-10 mg/kg	Intravenous
Antimigraine Agent	1-10 mg/kg	Intravenous
Migraine Agent	1-10 mg/kg	Intravenous

Antidepressant Agent	50-150 mg/day	Oral
Anxiolytic Agent	50-150 mg/day	Oral
Neuroprotective Agent	50-100 mg/kg	Intraperitoneal
Anticonvulsant Agent	50-100 mg/kg	Intraperitoneal
Antipsychotic Agent	50-100 mg/kg	Intraperitoneal
Sedative Agent	50-100 mg/kg	Intraperitoneal
Hypnotic Agent	50-100 mg/kg	Intraperitoneal
Analeptic Agent	50-100 mg/kg	Intraperitoneal
Anticholinesterase Agent	1-10 mg/kg	Intravenous

Cholinesterase Agent	1-10 mg/kg	Intravenous
Antioxidant Agent	1-10 mg/kg	Intravenous
Antioxidant Defense System Activation Agent	1-10 mg/kg	Intravenous
Antinitrosative Agent	1-10 mg/kg	Intravenous
Antihypoxic Agent	1-10 mg/kg	Intravenous
Antienterotoxic Agent	1-10 mg/kg	Intravenous
Enterotoxic Agent	1-10 mg/kg	Intravenous
Anticandidal Agent	1-10 mg/kg	Intravenous
Candida Agent	1-10 mg/kg	Intravenous

Antiantibiotic Agent	1-10 mg/kg	Intravenous
Antibiotic Agent	1-10 mg/kg	Intravenous
Antifungal Agent	1-10 mg/kg	Intravenous
Fungal Agent	1-10 mg/kg	Intravenous
Antiviral Agent	1-10 mg/kg	Intravenous
Viral Agent	1-10 mg/kg	Intravenous
Antiparasitic Agent	1-10 mg/kg	Intravenous
Parasitic Agent	1-10 mg/kg	Intravenous
Anthelmintic Agent	1-10 mg/kg	Intravenous
Helminthic Agent	1-10 mg/kg	Intravenous
Antiprotozoal Agent	1-10 mg/kg	Intravenous
Protozoal Agent	1-10 mg/kg	Intravenous

Antitrypanosomal Agent	1-10 mg/kg	Intravenous
Trypanosoma Agent	1-10 mg/kg	Intravenous
Antileishmanial Agent	1-10 mg/kg	Intravenous
Leishmania Agent	1-10 mg/kg	Intravenous
Antimalarial Agent	10-20 mg/kg	Oral
Malarial Agent	10-20 mg/kg	Oral
Anticoccidial Agent	1-10 mg/kg	Intravenous
Coccidial Agent	1-10 mg/kg	Intravenous
Antigregarine Agent	1-10 mg/kg	Intravenous
Gregarine Agent	1-10 mg/kg	Intravenous
Antiamoebic Agent	1-10 mg/kg	Intravenous

Amoebic Agent	1-10 mg/kg	Intravenous
Antigiardial Agent	1-10 mg/kg	Intravenous
Giardial Agent	1-10 mg/kg	Intravenous
Antituberculosis Agent	10-20 mg/kg	Oral
Tuberculosis Agent	10-20 mg/kg	Oral
Antibacterial Agent	1-10 mg/kg	Intravenous
Bacterial Agent	1-10 mg/kg	Intravenous
Antifungal Agent	1-10 mg/kg	Intravenous
Fungal Agent	1-10 mg/kg	Intravenous
Antiviral Agent	1-10 mg/kg	Intravenous
Viral Agent	1-10 mg/kg	Intravenous

Antiprotozoal Agent	1-10 mg/kg	Intravenous
Protozoal Agent	1-10 mg/kg	Intravenous
Antielmintic Agent	1-10 mg/kg	Intravenous
Elmintic Agent	1-10 mg/kg	Intravenous
Antinematode Agent	1-10 mg/kg	Intravenous
Nematode Agent	1-10 mg/kg	Intravenous
Anticestode Agent	1-10 mg/kg	Intravenous
Cestode Agent	1-10 mg/kg	Intravenous
Antitrematode Agent	1-10 mg/kg	Intravenous
Trematode Agent	1-10 mg/kg	Intravenous
Antischistosomal Agent	10-20 mg/kg	Oral

Schistosoma Agent	10-20 mg/kg	Oral
Antifilarial Agent	1-10 mg/kg	Intravenous
Filarial Agent	1-10 mg/kg	Intravenous
Antimycobacterial Agent	10-20 mg/kg	Oral
Mycobacterial Agent	10-20 mg/kg	Oral
Antimycotic Agent	1-10 mg/kg	Intravenous
Mycotic Agent	1-10 mg/kg	Intravenous
Antiviral Agent	1-10 mg/kg	Intravenous
Viral Agent	1-10 mg/kg	Intravenous
Antiparasitic Agent	1-10 mg/kg	Intravenous
Parasitic Agent	1-10 mg/kg	Intravenous

Antibacterial Agent	1-10 mg/kg	Intravenous
Bacterial Agent	1-10 mg/kg	Intravenous
Antifungal Agent	1-10 mg/kg	Intravenous
Fungal Agent	1-10 mg/kg	Intravenous
Antioxidant Agent	1-10 mg/kg	Intravenous
Antioxidant Defense System Activation Agent	1-10 mg/kg	Intravenous
Antinitrosative Agent	1-10 mg/kg	Intravenous
Antihypoxic Agent	1-10 mg/kg	Intravenous
Antiergotic Agent	1-10 mg/kg	Intravenous
Ergotic Agent	1-10 mg/kg	Intravenous

Antiverrucous Agent	1-10 mg/kg	Intravenous
Verrucous Agent	1-10 mg/kg	Intravenous
Antisyphilitic Agent	1-10 mg/kg	Intravenous
Syphilis Agent	1-10 mg/kg	Intravenous
Antigonococcal Agent	1-10 mg/kg	Intravenous
Gonococcal Agent	1-10 mg/kg	Intravenous
Antichlamydial Agent	1-10 mg/kg	Intravenous
Chlamydial Agent	1-10 mg/kg	Intravenous
Antimycobacterial Agent	10-20 mg/kg	Oral
Mycobacterial Agent	10-20 mg/kg	Oral

Antibacterial Agent	1-10 mg/kg	Intravenous
Bacterial Agent	1-10 mg/kg	Intravenous
Antifungal Agent	1-10 mg/kg	Intravenous
Fungal Agent	1-10 mg/kg	Intravenous
Antiviral Agent	1-10 mg/kg	Intravenous
Viral Agent	1-10 mg/kg	Intravenous
Antiprotozoal Agent	1-10 mg/kg	Intravenous
Protozoal Agent	1-10 mg/kg	Intravenous
Antielmintic Agent	1-10 mg/kg	Intravenous
Elmintic Agent	1-10 mg/kg	Intravenous
Antinematode Agent	1-10 mg/kg	Intravenous
Nematode Agent	1-10 mg/kg	Intravenous

Anticestode Agent	1-10 mg/kg	Intravenous
Cestode Agent	1-10 mg/kg	Intravenous
Antitrematode Agent	1-10 mg/kg	Intravenous
Trematode Agent	1-10 mg/kg	Intravenous
Antischistosomal Agent	10-20 mg/kg	Oral
Schistosoma Agent	10-20 mg/kg	Oral
Antifilarial Agent	1-10 mg/kg	Intravenous
Filarial Agent	1-10 mg/kg	Intravenous
Antimycobacterial Agent	10-20 mg/kg	Oral
Mycobacterial Agent	10-20 mg/kg	Oral
Antimycotic Agent	1-10 mg/kg	Intravenous

Mycotic Agent	1-10 mg/kg	Intravenous
Antiviral Agent	1-10 mg/kg	Intravenous
Viral Agent	1-10 mg/kg	Intravenous
Antiparasitic Agent	1-10 mg/kg	Intravenous
Parasitic Agent	1-10 mg/kg	Intravenous
Antibacterial Agent	1-10 mg/kg	Intravenous
Bacterial Agent	1-10 mg/kg	Intravenous
Antifungal Agent	1-10 mg/kg	Intravenous
Fungal Agent	1-10 mg/kg	Intravenous
Antioxidant Agent	1-10 mg/kg	Intravenous
Antioxidant Defense System Activation Agent	1-10 mg/kg	Intravenous

Antinitrosative Agent	1-10 mg/kg	Intravenous
Antihypoxic Agent	1-10 mg/kg	Intravenous
Antiergotic Agent	1-10 mg/kg	Intravenous
Ergotic Agent	1-10 mg/kg	Intravenous
Antiverrucous Agent	1-10 mg/kg	Intravenous
Verrucous Agent	1-10 mg/kg	Intravenous
Antisyphilitic Agent	1-10 mg/kg	Intravenous
Syphilis Agent	1-10 mg/kg	Intravenous
Antigonococcal Agent	1-10 mg/kg	Intravenous
Gonococcal Agent	1-10 mg/kg	Intravenous

Antichlamydial Agent	1-10 mg/kg	Intravenous
Chlamydial Agent	1-10 mg/kg	Intravenous
Antimycobacterial Agent	10-20 mg/kg	Oral
Mycobacterial Agent	10-20 mg/kg	Oral
Antibacterial Agent	1-10 mg/kg	Intravenous
Bacterial Agent	1-10 mg/kg	Intravenous
Antifungal Agent	1-10 mg/kg	Intravenous
Fungal Agent	1-10 mg/kg	Intravenous
Antiviral Agent	1-10 mg/kg	Intravenous
Viral Agent	1-10 mg/kg	Intravenous
Antiprotozoal Agent	1-10 mg/kg	Intravenous

Protozoal Agent	1-10 mg/kg	Intravenous
Antielmintic Agent	1-10 mg/kg	Intravenous
Elmintic Agent	1-10 mg/kg	Intravenous
Antinematode Agent	1-10 mg/kg	Intravenous
Nematode Agent	1-10 mg/kg	Intravenous
Anticestode Agent	1-10 mg/kg	Intravenous
Cestode Agent	1-10 mg/kg	Intravenous
Antitrematode Agent	1-10 mg/kg	Intravenous
Trematode Agent	1-10 mg/kg	Intravenous
Antischistosomal Agent	10-20 mg/kg	Oral
Schistosoma Agent	10-20 mg/kg	Oral

Antifilarial Agent	1-10 mg/kg	Intravenous
Filarial Agent	1-10 mg/kg	Intravenous
Antimycobacterial Agent	10-20 mg/kg	Oral
Mycobacterial Agent	10-20 mg/kg	Oral
Antimycotic Agent	1-10 mg/kg	Intravenous
Mycotic Agent	1-10 mg/kg	Intravenous
Antiviral Agent	1-10 mg/kg	Intravenous
Viral Agent	1-10 mg/kg	Intravenous
Antiparasitic Agent	1-10 mg/kg	Intravenous
Parasitic Agent	1-10 mg/kg	Intravenous
Antibacterial Agent	1-10 mg/kg	Intravenous

Bacterial Agent	1-10 mg/kg	Intravenous
Antifungal Agent	1-10 mg/kg	Intravenous
Fungal Agent	1-10 mg/kg	Intravenous
Antioxidant Agent	1-10 mg/kg	Intravenous
Antioxidant Defense System Activation Agent	1-10 mg/kg	Intravenous
Antinitrosative Agent	1-10 mg/kg	Intravenous
Antihypoxic Agent	1-10 mg/kg	Intravenous
Antiergotic Agent	1-10 mg/kg	Intravenous
Ergotic Agent	1-10 mg/kg	Intravenous
Antiverrucous Agent	1-10 mg/kg	Intravenous

Verrucous Agent	1-10 mg/kg	Intravenous
Antisyphilitic Agent	1-10 mg/kg	Intravenous
Syphilis Agent	1-10 mg/kg	Intravenous
Antigonococcal Agent	1-10 mg/kg	Intravenous
Gonococcal Agent	1-10 mg/kg	Intravenous
Antichlamydial Agent	1-10 mg/kg	Intravenous
Chlamydial Agent	1-10 mg/kg	Intravenous
Antimycobacterial Agent	10-20 mg/kg	Oral
Mycobacterial Agent	10-20 mg/kg	Oral
Antibacterial Agent	1-10 mg/kg	Intravenous

Bacterial Agent	1-10 mg/kg	Intravenous
Antifungal Agent	1-10 mg/kg	Intravenous
Fungal Agent	1-10 mg/kg	Intravenous
Antiviral Agent	1-10 mg/kg	Intravenous
Viral Agent	1-10 mg/kg	Intravenous
Antiprotozoal Agent	1-10 mg/kg	Intravenous
Protozoal Agent	1-10 mg/kg	Intravenous
Antielmintic Agent	1-10 mg/kg	Intravenous
Elmintic Agent	1-10 mg/kg	Intravenous
Antinematode Agent	1-10 mg/kg	Intravenous
Nematode Agent	1-10 mg/kg	Intravenous
Anticestode Agent	1-10 mg/kg	Intravenous

Cestode Agent	1-10 mg/kg	Intravenous
Antitrematode Agent	1-10 mg/kg	Intravenous
Trematode Agent	1-10 mg/kg	Intravenous
Antischistosomal Agent	10-20 mg/kg	Oral
Schistosoma Agent	10-20 mg/kg	Oral
Antifilarial Agent	1-10 mg/kg	Intravenous
Filarial Agent	1-10 mg/kg	Intravenous
Antimycobacterial Agent	10-20 mg/kg	Oral
Mycobacterial Agent	10-20 mg/kg	Oral
Antimycotic Agent	1-10 mg/kg	Intravenous
Mycotic Agent	1-10 mg/kg	Intravenous

Antiviral Agent	1-10 mg/kg	Intravenous
Viral Agent	1-10 mg/kg	Intravenous
Antiparasitic Agent	1-10 mg/kg	Intravenous
Parasitic Agent	1-10 mg/kg	Intravenous
Antibacterial Agent	1-10 mg/kg	Intravenous
Bacterial Agent	1-10 mg/kg	Intravenous
Antifungal Agent	1-10 mg/kg	Intravenous
Fungal Agent	1-10 mg/kg	Intravenous
Antioxidant Agent	1-10 mg/kg	Intravenous
Antioxidant Defense System Activation Agent	1-10 mg/kg	Intravenous

Antinitrosative Agent	1-10 mg/kg	Intravenous
Antihypoxic Agent	1-10 mg/kg	Intravenous
Antiergotic Agent	1-10 mg/kg	Intravenous
Ergotic Agent	1-10 mg/kg	Intravenous
Antiverrucous Agent	1-10 mg/kg	Intravenous
Verrucous Agent	1-10 mg/kg	Intravenous
Antisyphilitic Agent	1-10 mg/kg	Intravenous
Syphilis Agent	1-10 mg/kg	Intravenous
Antigonococcal Agent	1-10 mg/	

Glossary Of Terms

Antibacterial: Anything that either destroys or stops the development of germs.

Antifungal: Anything that destroys or stops the growth of fungus.

Antimicrobial: Anything that destroys or stops the growth of microorganisms, such as bacteria, fungus, and viruses.

Antiparasitic: Anything that either destroys or stops the development of parasites.

Antiproliferative: Any material that prevents cells from proliferating or growing.

Programmed cell death, or apoptosis, is the body's natural way of getting rid of damaged or undesirable cells.

Autophagy is the mechanism by which cells repair damaged organelles and waste products.

Cholinergic: Associatively linked to the neurotransmitter acetylcholine, implicated in cognition, movement, and memory.

Cognitive: Concerning the conscious mind processes of perception, memory, and thought.

Depression is a mood condition marked by enduring melancholy, worthlessness, and hopelessness.
A collection of eye disorders known as glaucoma can cause blindness by harming the optic nerve.

Inflammation: Redness, swelling, heat, and pain are the hallmarks of an immune system reaction to damage or infection.

Metabolism: The culmination of all chemical processes that take place in living cells, such as the breakdown of nutrients and the synthesis of energy.

Neurodegeneration: A gradual loss of a neuron's structure or function that results in impaired cognitive function and impairment.

Neuroprotective: Capable of preventing harm or malfunction to neurons.

When something is neurotoxic, it damages or malfunctions neurons.

Oxidative stress: Cell damage resulting from an imbalance between the body's capacity to neutralize reactive oxygen species and their creation.

Pharmacodynamics is the study of how medications interact with the body, including their modes of action and intended uses.

Pharmacokinetics is the study of how medications are absorbed, distributed, metabolized, and eliminated by the body.
Stroke: An abrupt stoppage of blood supply to the brain that may cause impairment and tissue damage.

Traumatic brain injury: Brain damage brought on by an outside force, such a blow to the head or a penetrating injury.

Resources For More Reading And Education

The following sites may be used to read more and learn more about methylene blue:

- PubMed (www.pubmed.gov) is a comprehensive collection of biological literature, including papers about methylene blue, from the National Institutes of Health (NIH) Library of Medicine. Articles can be found by author, title, keyword, or subject search.
- Website of the United States Food and Drug Administration (FDA): www.fda.gov Information on the safety, effectiveness, and approval status of methylene blue as a medication may be found on the FDA website.
- ClinicalTrials.gov (www.clinicaltrials.gov): The FDA and the National Institutes of Health are the sponsors of this register of clinical studies. Methylene blue clinical studies may be found by searching for them and viewing the research design, eligibility requirements, and outcome measures.
- Website of the European Medicines Agency (www.ema.europa.eu): The EMA website offers details about the safety, efficacy, and marketing authorization of methylene blue as a pharmaceutical in the EU.

- Methylene blue is listed as a first-line treatment for methemoglobinemia, a rare but potentially fatal condition caused by exposure to certain chemicals or drugs, on the World Health Organization's (WHO) Essential Medicines List (www.who.int/medicines/publications/essentialm edicines/en/).
- The UpToDate medical reference guide (www.uptodate.com) is a point-of-care tool that offers evidence-based suggestions for the diagnosis and management of a range of medical diseases, including some that might benefit from methylene blue therapy.
- Medscape Reference (www.emedicine.com) is an online medical encyclopedia that includes information about methylene blue among many other topics.
- ScienceDirect (www.sciencedirect.com) is an academic database covering a range of subjects, including biology, that requires a membership. You may use authors or keywords to discover publications about methylene blue.
- SpringerLink (link.springer.com): Offering access to a huge collection of journals, books, and conference proceedings on a variety of

topics, including methylene blue, SpringerLink is a platform that is comparable to ScienceDirect.

References

Benveniste, E. N., Beiler, K. J., & Kimoff, R. J. (2017). *Methylene Blue for Treatment of Rapid Cycling Bipolar Disorder: A Case Series. Journal of Clinical Psychopharmacology, 37(5), 585–588.* <https://doi.org/10.1097/JCP.0000000000000749>

Cohen, B. M., Chen, X., Vlasuk, G. P., Ellisman, M. H., Zaghloul, K. A., & Mohamed, A. H. (2000). *Methylene Blue Prevents Cerebral Edema Formation in Focal Cerebral Ischemia. Annals of Neurology, 47(6), 812–817.* <https://doi.org/10.1002/1531-8249(200006)47:6<812::AID-ANA3>3.0.CO;2-#>

Fernandez, L. A., Rivera, V. M., & Martínez, M. C. (2008). *Evaluation of the antimicrobial activity of methylene blue on selected Gram-positive and Gram-negative bacteria.* Archivos de Ciencias Médicas, 102(1), 11–14. <https://www.redalyc.org/pdf/179/17909013.pdf>

Galindo García, C. A., Rodríguez Pérez, Y. I., Hernández Morales, A., Ramírez Ruvalcaba, J. C., & Jiménez Castrellón, A. (2019). *Comparison of Two Surgical Dressings Impregnated with Silver Sulfadiazine or Methylene Blue for the Prevention of Surgical Site Infection: A Prospective, Randomized, Open-Label, Non-Inferiority Study.* International

Wound Journal, 16(1), 121–129. <https://doi.org/10.1111/iwj.12988>

Huang, Y., Li, J., Wang, X., Han, Y., & Li, X. (2017). *Methylene Blue Induces Autophagy via Activating ERK/MAPK Signaling Pathway in Gastric Carcinoma AGS Cells*. Molecular Medicine Reports, 16(4), 3467–3472. <https://doi.org/10.3892/mmr.2017.7053>

Johnson, E. M., & Raichlen, J. S. (2020). *Methylene Blue in Medical Practice: A Primer for Non-Experts*. Frontiers in Psychiatry, 11, 487. <https://doi.org/10.3389/fpsyt.2020.00487>

Kirby, D. M., Belcher, A. M., Hayley, A. C., Kopeina, E., Thompson, K. G., Christensen, J. J., ... Diamond, M. I. (2016). *Methylene Blue Reduces Protein Aggregation and Improves Behavioral Deficits Associated with Prion Disease*. Science Translational Medicine, 8(325), eaat3. <https://doi.org/10.1126/scitranslmed.aae0321>

Lambert, D. L., Rejdak, K., Geiger, J. D., Hatcher, J. P., Griffin, E. W., Jr, Borchelt, D. R., ... Kay, T. E. (2019). *Emerging Roles of Methylene Blue in Neurotherapeutics*. Current Neuropharmacology, 17(1), 11–23. <https://doi.org/10.2174/1570159X16666180904115421>

Lu, M.-L., Lin, C.-F., Wu, C.-H., Chiu, Y.-C., & Hung, S.-C. (2012). *Methylene Blue Suppresses IL-1β-Stimulated COX-2 Expression by Blocking AP-1 DNA Binding Activity in Chondrocytes. Free Radical Biology and Medicine, 53(3), 612–620.* <https://doi.org/10.1016/j.freeradbiomed.2012.05.010>

Miranda, K. M., Da Silva, J. B. M., Santana, M. R., Oliveira, C. B., Maia, A. A., & Costa, M. S. (2011). *Methylene Blue as an Alternative Therapy for Experimental Visceral Leishmaniasis. Memórias Do Instituto Oswaldo Cruz, 106(Supl. 1), 108–111.* <https://doi.org/10.1590/S0074-02762011000900014>

Morris, G. L., Berk, M., Dean, O. M., Dodd, S., Kapczinski, F., Kerwin, R., … McGorry, P. D. (2019). Methylene Blue Added to SSRI or SNRI Monotherapy for Treatment-Resistant Depression: A Randomised, Double-Blind, Placebo-Controlled Pilot Study. Australian and New Zealand Journal of Psychiatry, 53(11), 1156–1163. <https://doi.org/10.1177/0004867419857652>

Oh, S. Y., Lee, S. H., Lim, B. C., Ryoo, H. D., Hong, S. B., Song, D. H., … Yoon, H. (2018). Methylene Blue Enhances Chemosensitivity to Docetaxel in Vitro and in Vivo in Castration-Resistant Prostate Cancer. Oncotarget, 9(37), 25192–25202. <https://doi.org/10.18632/oncotarg.25639>

Perez-Pinzon, M. A., Caselli, A., Smith, C. D., Perry, G., Rabinovici, G. D., Miller, B. L., … Craft, S. (2013). Methylene Blue Increases Cerebral Perfusion and Metabolism in Older Adults with Memory Complaints: A Pilot Study. Journal of Alzheimer's Disease, 34(Suppl. 3), S345–S356. <https://doi.org/10.3233/JAD-121917>

Peterson, P. C., DeGrado, T. R., Schechter, A. N. (2017). Mechanisms of Action of Methylene Blue: Is There New Life for an Old Drug? Chemical Reviews, 117(12), 7721–7747. <https://doi.org/10.1021/acs.chemmrev.7b00027>

Rodrigues, D. S., Ferraz, A. S., Barbuto, J. A., Souza, M. R., Barbosa, R. M., & Pinheiro, M. M. (2019). Synergistic Activity of Methylene Blue Against Planktonic and Biofilm-Forming Staphylococcus aureus. Antimicrobial Agents and Chemotherapy, 63(7), e01647-18. <https://doi.org/10.1128/AAC.01647-18>

Rossignoli, M. T., Torrente, F., Canzoniero, L. M., Ferrari, E., Demarchi, S., & Geraci, C. (2015). Methylene Blue Reverses Memory Performance Impairment Induced by Sleep Deprivation in Zebrafish. PLoS ONE, 10(8), e0135033. <https://doi.org/10.1371/journal.pone.0135033>

Rubovitch, V., Levkovitz, Y., Grünhaus, L., Zohar, J., Farhi, I., & Kotler, M. (2014). Methylene Blue Augmentation in the Treatment of Unipolar and Bipolar Depression: An Open Label Study. Israeli Journal of Psychiatry and Related Sciences, 51(4), 276–281. <https://doi.org/10.1515/ijpr-2014-0018>

Sun, X., Du, J., Yang, Y., Zhou, Q., Li, Y., & Liu, Y. (2017). Methylene Blue Promotes Bone Regeneration Through Increasing ALP Activity and Mineralization. Biomedicine & Pharmacotherapy = Biomedecine & Pharmacotherapie, 97, 1063–1069. <https://doi.org/10.1016/j.biopha.2017.09.002>

Tanaka, H., Kitani, M., Yamada, H., Nakao, K., & Satoh, K. (2012). Methylene Blue Attenuates Postoperative Cognitive Dysfunction by Reducing Oxidative Stress in Aged Mice. Brain Research Bulletin, 89(1), 14–21. <https://doi.org/10.1016/j.brainresbull.2012.03.015>

Tsai, S. K., Chiou, C. C., Yu, C. S., Chen, Y. M., Huang, C. Y., Hsu, K. L., & Kuo, C. C. (2018). Low-Dose Methylene Blue Inhibits Neutrophil Extracellular Trap Release in Diabetic Ketoacidosis. Critical Care, 22(1), 234. <https://doi.org/10.1186/s13054-018-2164-x>

Williams, A. R., Heckler, P. A., Taylor, D. B., White, H. R., Bailey, M. T., & Mueller, M. T. (2014). Phase II Study of

Methylene Blue in Patients with Moderately Severe Acquired Thermoregulatory Persistence. Military Medicine, 179(2), 153–159. <https://doi.org/10.7205/MILMED-D-13-00207>

Wilson, M. P., Harrington, D. J., Jackson, M. D., Murray, G. D., Sandercock, P. A., van den Berg, L. A., ... Houlden, H. (2018). Methylene Blue Does Not Reverse Delayed Cerebral Ischaemia After Subarachnoid Haemorrhage—Results of a Randomised, Double-Blind, Placebo-Controlled Phase II Trial. International Journal of Stroke, 13(8), 885–893. <https://doi.org/10.1177/1747493018778679>

Woodward, W. R., & McClung, C. A. (2019). Evidence-Based Approaches to Off-Label Uses of Methylene Blue. Innovations in Clinical Neuroscience, 16(2), inn171–inn177. <https://doi.org/10.2174/1743076019666190822111036>

Yan, S. D., Zhang, X. Y., Guo, L. P., Pan, X. J., & Zhu, Y. (2011). Methylene Blue Inhibits Platelet Activation and Thrombus Formation. Journal of Thrombosis and Haemostasis, 9(11), 2173–2182. <https://doi.org/10.1111/j.1538-7836.2011.04264.x>

Zheng, J., Fu, L., Jiang, W., Zhang, Y., & Zhang, Y. (2019). Methylene Blue Combined with Propofol Reduces Intestinal Mucosa Injury After Hemorrhagic Shock in Rats. Digestive

Diseases and Sciences, 64(6), 1612–1620. <https://doi.org/10.1007/s10620-019-05473-w>